Your Skin:

AN OWNER'S GUIDE

D0062725

YOUR
SKIN
...An Owner's Guide

JOSEPH P. BARK, M.D.

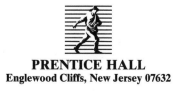

PRENTICE HALL
Englewood Cliffs, New Jersey 07632

Prentice Hall International (UK) Limited, *London*
Prentice Hall of Australia Pty. Limited, *Sydney*
Prentice Hall Canada, Inc., *Toronto*
Prentice Hall Hispanoamericana, S.A., *Mexico*
Prentice Hall of India Private Limited, *New Delhi*
Prentice Hall of Japan, Inc., *Tokyo*
Simon & Schuster Asia Pte. Ltd., *Singapore*
Editora Prentice Hall do Brasil, Ltda., *Rio de Janeiro*

10 9 8 7 6 5 4 3 2 1

Library of Congress Cataloging-in-Publication Data

Bark, Joseph P.
    Your skin : an owner's guide / Joseph P. Bark
        p.   cm.
    Includes index.
    ISBN 0-13-199663-0
    1. Skin—Care and hygiene. 2. Dermatology—
Popular works. I. Title.
RL87.B353   1995
616.5—dc20   95-16749
                                                                    CIP

ISBN 0-13-199663-0

Prentice Hall
Career & Personal Development
Englewood Cliffs, NJ 07632

A Simon & Schuster Company

Printed in the United States of America

For Lin—The adventure, the beauty, the intellect, the playfulness, the laughter, and the softness in my life...

Acknowledgments

I would like to thank Donna E. Roth, M.D. for her enlightened update on the science of laser treatment of the skin. Dr. Roth, a master diagnostician and dermatologist has made each of my days more exciting in the practice of dermatology.

John L. Buker, M.D., has written the section on Mohs Surgery and treatment of skin cancers. Having come to us from the National Naval Medical Center in Bethesda, after eight years as Chairman of Dermatologic Surgery, he has shown us true art in surgery on countless occasions.

To Rhonda Waller-Smith, my personal assistant and right hand, I owe much appreciation. Her steady hand has helped guide me through this project with veteran skill, and her excellence and insistence on accuracy have been the guidepost of this effort.

To Rosalie Heacock, whose gracious spouse and associate Jim Heacock encouraged this project, I give my love and respectful sympathy. We shall miss Jim intensely.

Preface

Sometime late in my third year at the University of Kentucky College of Medicine I was working in the neonatal intensive care unit. As I was trying to insert a small butterfly needle into a scalp vein of an infant, a fellow in a bright sport coat walked leisurely into the neonatal unit, put on a sterile gown, and came into the "baby brig," as we called it. He stepped up to my side and announced, "I'm Marsh in dermatology. Is the Saunders baby here?"

"Yes," I said, pointing to the next incubator, "That's him over there." Dr. Glenn Marsh strolled over and very gently picked up a tiny leg with a bulbous red spot on the thigh. I remembered seeing it on rounds earlier in the day.

"Hemangioma," he said. "No sweat!"

"You mean you can fix it?" I asked, as I pulled out my second try at the scalp vein.

Marsh glanced over his shoulder and said, "God'll fix that one, Doctor Bark," glancing at my name tag. "Most of them go away without any treatment at all."

"Fascinating!" I said, as I prepared to stick my diminutive patient again. "We thought he'd be in for long hours under the knife!"

"Nope. They fade beautifully almost every time! You ought to think about dermatology. I think you'd find it very interesting!" And, in fact, the dermatology elective I took in Dr. Marsh's private office the next year introduced me to my career of answering questions about the skin.

Later, in my residency in dermatology, I found myself faced with a quizzical look on a patient named John with white spots on his face. I was explaining to John that he had a common problem of middle age. It was sebaceous hyperplasia. I went on to explain that sometimes the sebaceous glands of the face underwent hypertrophy during the aging process.

With my every word John's face showed more and more confusion, until finally he said, "Listen, Doctor, have you been talking to me for the last five minutes? If so," he said, "you'd better give me a few years to go to medical school before you continue this explanation. Then I might understand it!"

I decided then and there to launch a campaign to make medicine more easily understandable to those who matter the most: my patients.

Since then I've found that one of the greatest thrills in medicine is the thanks of a patient who has had a problem explained in words that can be understood. It seems that we doctors just don't seem to take the time to do that anymore. I wish all doctors would realize that "enlarged oil glands accompanying middle age" sounds infinitely better than "hyperplastic pilosebaceous follicles."

So it has become a hobby for me, you see, a sort of constant challenge, to explain things to my patients in words they understand.

I don't always succeed. For instance, a young woman named Mary came to me one day with a vaginal yeast infection and a very itchy discharge. After her examination I was interested to find out if she and her husband were ping-ponging this infectious yeast back and forth, so I asked her, "Is your husband circumcised?" A quizzical look followed. So, not wanting to give her more time to be embarrassed, I further questioned, "Well, does he have a foreskin on his penis?" Mary mumbled a terse word or two I could not hear. We both squirmed a little, and I realized I was in trouble.

I decided I could either drop the subject and miss a possible source of contagion (along with the possible embarrassment), or I could pursue it further. Unfortunately, I pursued it. I next held up a thumb as if to represent a penis and slowly encircled it with my index finger as if to demonstrate where a foreskin might be located. "Does he have a foreskin on his penis?" I asked, more emphatically.

Mary, growing livid with my pursuit of the subject, glowered straight at me and said, "Doctor, I just do not know!"

I decided it was time to break off the inquiry. I felt sure that if he had had that infection under his foreskin he would eventually have found his way to a physician for treatment. Sometimes the doctor can't win no matter what words are used.

You can see that medical explanations can quickly get out of hand. But I've tried to break down the medical terminology and vital dermatologic information in this book into terms that are understandable to those outside the medical community. Realize, though, that in a single volume I can really attack only the most prevalent problems involved in dermatologic care.

Since the skin is the largest and most visible of all the body's organs, the science of dermatology is one of the oldest of all medical sciences.

In the last fifty years, dermatology has acquired a great deal of respect from the general medical community for dealing with a vast array of cutaneous illnesses unknown to ordinary physicians during their medical training.

Because I have spent my professional career answering questions, even traveling all over the country speaking about skin care, I have decided to write down some of the most important questions dermatologists are asked and give clearly understandable answers to these questions.

Introduction

The skin is your body's largest organ! And to think that this is true
for every human being, and yet we generally know so little about it,
nor do we have to think much about its care! This magnificent
organ, the body's protective suit, air conditioner, subject of a thousand poems and a million caresses, essentially takes care of itself. It
is, in fact, a rare instance when we have to think of it at all, except,
as they say, "when something is wrong with it." But, when it is, we all
need help in analyzing and treating or seeking treatment for the
noisome diseases of the skin, and we should all be aware that some
skin diseases are much, much more than just noisome.

But this is a highly specialized field. And the fact that skin is so
close to us and our eyes is the reason why so many topical preparations are available for its treatment (or mistreatment). We clearly
need some source for good skin advice, and lacking an appointment for the dermatologist's advice directly, I have chosen to try to
give you the practical, everyday advice for proper skin health and
treatment of minor skin afflictions, as well as advice on when to
actually go see the dermatologist for more serious problems.

You should use this book as you would an encyclopedia. In
fact, that is why we call it an owner's guide. You should look up your
symptom or condition in the index and read all about it and the
possible diseases with which it could be associated. Then, I will
often tell you about ways you can approach treatment at home,
preparations that are safe to buy over the counter, or when to go see
the doctor.

You can also use this book to actually *help* your dermatologist.
For instance, many of my patients have brought books and popular
lay magazines into the office in which they have accurately spotted
their diagnoses! This is often useful for your doctor, especially if the
book or article puts your symptoms into words better than perhaps
you could have. Often your doctor will thank you for helping
him/her in the diagnosis of your problem, and this expedites treat-

ment. So, if you spot a condition in this book that resembles yours, take the book to your dermatologist and *show* it to him/her.

Lastly, pay special attention to the sections in this book which refer to sun damage and the skin. As our ozone layer thins and develops holes allowing more intense sun damage in years to come, we will all need the best possible sun protection. Avoidance is the best protection you can get, and sunscreens are the next best.

I have listed many brand names of products in this book which are placed here so you can actually use the book to help your skin on a day-to-day basis. I have no interest in these products whatsoever, except that they help your skin and have been found efficacious in this regard.

YOUR SKIN DOCTOR

Dermatologists are indeed medical doctors or doctors of osteopathy as well. They've completed four years of medical school to get their medical degree, a year of internship, and three years of residency.

But most dermatologists are pretty strict at sticking to the specialty for which we're trained: skin medicine. That's not to say that, in an emergency, we wouldn't treat you for something else, but as a rule, your family doctor should handle your sore throat and other general medical problems.

If a problem can be seen or felt, it can be initially evaluated by a dermatologist. That does not mean that all such problems can be handled by the dermatologist, but it's certainly an excellent starting point if you are concerned about any skin spot or symptom. Itching, for instance, which is usually a reaction to external irritants, can also be a sign of diabetes and many other internal diseases, such as hidden malignancies and infections.

Your dermatologist, like any other physician, will establish basic information about your background through the use of your medical record. He or she will question you about the history of your problem, including significant past and social history, and will perform an examination of the skin and other systems pertinent to your complaint.

To clarify the diagnosis of difficult rashes, many dermatologists are equipped to perform laboratory tests such as fungus cultures and various other stains and microscopic preparations right in their offices.

Dermatology is a peculiarly mixed specialty, having medical and surgical modes. Almost every dermatologist does minor surgery, and many do dermabrasions, minor cosmetic surgery, and minor plastic surgical procedures.

I hate to hedge on the question of costs. However, dermatologic costs are found to vary greatly among practitioners and more so among various areas of the country where fee schedules have been established. A guesstimate, however, is that initial office fees for a dermatologist will run in the $50 to $75 bracket; surgical charges, injections, and medications will add to this figure.

I suggest to anyone who has questions about charges that he or she talk to the doctor frankly about this before procedures are done or medication given.

In general, prescription medicines (both internal and topical) are more beneficial than over-the-counter preparations, because over-the-counter medicine companies cannot make their medicines strong enough to do as much good because of the risk of side effects. The fact that a medicine is dispensed by prescription means that there are certain risks or side effects that must be weighed against the benefits of using the medicine to clear a specific skin problem. This judgment is made by the physician, who then has the license to write the prescription and accepts responsibility for doing so.

So if you have used an over-the-counter medicine to treat a specific skin problem and it is not working, see a dermatologist for further guidance and possibly prescription medicines.

WHERE TO GO FOR HELP

If you want information about certain topics not mentioned in this book, consult your dermatologist. Ask your dermatologist for information sheets or handouts concerning your skin disease or condition. You can then refer to them for salient treatment points when you wish to recall them later. Call your dermatologist or write to:

The American Academy of Dermatology
PO Box 4014
Schaumburg, IL 60168-4014

HOW TO USE THIS BOOK

When you perceive a rash, a bump, a lump, or a symptom in or on your skin, it's time to start searching this book for your specific condition. I've tried to include most of the more common skin maladies so that you can find them easily and so you can see if there are remedies you can use for yourself or whether you must see a dermatologist. I suggest you use the extensive index contained in this book to find your specific problem. First try looking up the symptom, such as "pigmented skin lesions," or "moles," and/or the symptom involved, such as "itching." Many different conditions are indexed for ease in finding your specific problem. I suggest a once-over quick read through the book to start. If you do this conscientiously, you will really know more about dermatology than most general practitioners of medicine (unless they take the time to read it too, which they should do!).

Once you find the specific section that applies to you, you should read it a couple of times carefully to see if the advice contained therein really applies to you. If not, you should consider that you may need to actually visit the dermatologist, and you should not hesitate to do this as soon as you determine that need.

I suggest, if you find a disease or condition in this text that seems to apply to you, that you mark it with a sticky-note and *take this book into the doctor* and ask him or her if you could be on the right track. You will be amazed at how often you will have helped out the doctor (and sometimes even the dermatologist!) by bringing the correct list of diagnoses to the fore.

Contents

One

BASIC CARE AND MAINTENANCE
1

Two

TROUBLESHOOTING
COMMON SKIN PROBLEMS
7

BASIC CARE
AND
MAINTENANCE

How Your Skin Works

As the body's largest organ, the skin is so prominent and all-encompassing that we often forget that it's there until we have a problem with it. But when you think about this magnificent suit we've been given to "cover our innards," it's no wonder that we generally ignore it—it renews itself and heals itself so well that it needs no more care than minimal cleanliness and repair from time to time.

The skin is our interface (connection) with the outside world. It is present on the body to prevent the portable sea that is our tissue fluid and blood from evaporating. In short, the skin supports life in many unperceived ways. Did you know, for example, that the skin is the most efficient air-conditioning system ever known? Blood flow through the skin is extremely effective in heat transfer to the outside environment from the internal one. Over the eons, the skin has developed evaporative and convective cooling to a fine art, so that the slightest change in our emotional state or ambient temperature causes subtle, nearly undetectable changes to control the temperature of our insides within an extremely narrow band.

Our eccrine, watery sweat glands secrete several liters of liquid daily that evaporates insensibly from our skins, taking the caloric heat of food and muscle metabolism with it into the air surrounding us. And if that weren't enough, the skin's blood vessels widen immediately upon these stresses so that convection currents can also expend heat into the environment.

On the other hand, if we didn't have many of the components of skin, we would die of cold exposure at the slightest insult. The skin's blood vessels clamp shut to preserve our core heat vital to life anytime we are exposed to cold. The skin's fat layer (although many wish they had *less* fat layer!) acts like a thick layer of insulation for the vital structures below. Without it we could simply not preserve our body heat. It's as simple as that.

Now think of the way the skin renews itself. It is a perfect suit covering the body, fitting every crevice, and as it ages it only sags a little—it never wears out, *never*! Every twenty-eight days we get an entirely new epidermis, from top to bottom! And a pool of nondividing cells is always at rest in the basement layers of the epidermis ready to take over the function of covering the body should they be needed. Even in old age (and this may be one of the *keys* to getting old) there is a population of resting young cells waiting to be released into the growth and proliferation phase. What if we could unlock these cells on *our* terms? Couldn't we stay younger looking almost indefinitely? Believe it or not, work such as this is currently under way. Regardless of how long it lasts, we must deal with the skin we have right now. That is the purpose of this book—to give you a plan of action and an instruction manual for a skin owner. Everyone needs directions on proper treatment of this complicated organ, and you are holding yours in your hand at this instant.

Basic Maintenance of Your Skin

Gentle soap and water, moisturizer, sunscreen, some Retin-A for resurfacing minor defects, and the knowledge of when to see the dermatologist. That's it!

Maybe you think I'm kidding, but you don't need all the magic miracle cures that so many companies are trying to sell you these days. "No one undergoes skin failure," to quote Dr. Al Kligman. So slathering on ten or twenty different (and expensive) products for some imagined reason is not sensible. Sensible care of your skin (basic maintenance) means the minimum you need to stay as cutaneously healthy as the next man or woman. And you see what you really need in the paragraph above.

Each of the items I mention above will be talked about in this book. Each item has its own place for discussion. The point to make right now is to stop heeding every commercial you hear about some new skin product that's supposed to perform some magical feat. There is no magic potion that will take care of all the problems with your skin. It doesn't exist.

The bottom line is that to understand good basic skin care you must determine first if you have any specific problems with your skin, treat them knowledgeably, and don't get involved in expensive noncures for nonproblems.

The Real Skin Secret Is You!

Soon you'll have all the information in your grasp to help your skin live a long, wrinkle-free, healthy, and beautiful life—so use it! You are the real secret to your skin health. You can make it all happen if you'll just follow a few simple tips to healthy skin.

During many of my talks for the American Cancer Society, people always ask, "How can I really give myself the 'best shot' at living without cancer?" It's a question that really sums up what everyone wants to know about a terrible menace. But that very useful question has been the basis around which I have constructed this book: "What are the skin secrets I need to know to keep my body's largest organ healthy and beautiful all my life?" Note: The question was not "What can my doctor do to keep my skin healthy?" We now live in a world where responsibility for acting on information is ours, once we have it.

Here are some vital rules to keep you healthy:

1. A baby's skin is extremely fragile—don't do anything to it that you don't find absolutely necessary. Use a mild soap and don't put medicated lotions and creams on an infant unless specifically ordered to do so by your pediatrician or dermatologist.

2. When your children's oil glands end their long hibernation in puberty, watch the child like a hawk. If you catch the acne process early, you may virtually save your children's social lives. Insist on a regular cleansing program with soap and water and demand early dermatologic care for any child with an acne problem.

3. Avoid sunlight! It's the single worst influence your skin will ever undergo. Just ask the 600,000 or so people (in the U.S. alone) who develop skin cancers every year. And don't forget to consider yourself an active member of my Tan Is Tacky Club. Use an SPF-15 sunscreen whenever you'll be exposed to the sun.

4. In my opinion, tanning parlors are a public menace. Remember that even the so-called safe systems of tanning beds can apparently cause problems as severe as cataracts, premature aging, skin cancer, and even changes in the immune system. Avoid them. Don't physically fry your beautiful skin.

5. Got something growing on you? Get it checked! Review the signs and symptoms of skin cancer at every opportunity. Procrastinating can allow benign lumps and bumps to get bigger and harder to remove. And for malignant problems of the skin, waiting too long can be fatal. Remember that skin cancers are easily cured if caught in time.

6. Finally, get yourself and your family a dermatologist. In the final analysis, your dermatologist is the professional who best knows how to diagnose and treat skin diseases—not the allergist, pediatrician, gynecologist, or internist—the dermatologist! Skin is a dermatologist's life! And with the vigilant help of your dermatologist, your skin will healthily last you all of yours!

TROUBLE-SHOOTING COMMON SKIN PROBLEMS

$\mathscr{A}cne$

THE WAR AGAINST ACNE—
A STRUGGLE TO SAVE FACE

Every month I see hundreds of teenagers who are battling their way through a desperate fight that, for some, will last for all their teen years and even beyond. That fight occurs as nature starts to create for them supple, adult skin lubricated and ready for the rest of their lives.

I've always felt it a shame that most people fail to realize how important a teenager's face is to him or her. Is it possible that they forget the struggles of being a teenager? I guess so, because day after day I see kids who won't talk, won't socialize, won't even look at me sometimes, because they're so ashamed of their appearance.

In fact, I'm sure that acne is one reason why I'm so dedicated to dermatology. As faces clear, I often see personalities blossom on subsequent office visits just like time-lapse pictures of an opening rose. What a delightful experience for a physician to see children climb out of the sadness that is acne.

The real problem with acne is delay—delay in talking over the situation with parents, and delay in seeking dermatologic help. Early help from a dermatologist for severe acne can save not only a youngster's skin but the psyche as well.

Acne is a disease that can last for years in some teens. It's a process in which the tiny tubes leading from the oil glands become completely or partially plugged. This results in back pressure on the oil glands themselves and trapping of bacteria. These bacteria are called *Propionibacterium acnes*. These *P. acnes* bacteria do not actually cause an infection, but the bacteria multiply within the oil gland, producing an enzyme called lipase that splits oil into very irritating substances called fatty acids. These cause irritation of the oil gland and eventual rupture of it, resulting in what appears as a red acne bump.

8

TREATMENTS

There are thousands of treatments for teenage complexion problems. Choosing the right ones from among the many over-the-counter and prescription products is the most important therapeutic dilemma in acne treatment. Let's look at a few types.

ANTIBIOTICS

There are reasons why dermatologists use each of the substances we will discuss. First of all, tetracycline is an excellent antibiotic that has been used in acne therapy for years. It has two functions. The first of these is to kill off the *P. acnes* bacteria. Happily, they are exquisitely sensitive to that medicine. Also, the tetracycline appears to be an inhibitor of the enzyme lipase, which causes rotting of the oil below the surface. In short, it's a bump stopper. If your dermatologist prescribes tetracycline for your acne, make sure you let him or her know if you are on a birth control pill. Some pills' effectiveness is decreased by tetracycline.

ASTRINGENTS

Several cosmetic companies sell "oil control" liquids to be put on after astringents and before makeup. These products are supposed to inhibit the appearance of shine on the skin for a long time. While not actually harmful, they can cause problems. There's really nothing that can stop oil from being secreted by the skin (that is, with the exception of Accutane, the new acne medicine that actually does stop it). So you're really left with removing the oil as it forms with astringents, or by covering up the oil with absorbent powders. These products are not harmful; they just don't really do what they claim to do. They remove surface oil only.

BENZOYL PEROXIDE

Topical benzoyl peroxide has several uses in acne. Some consider its main function one of a drying and peeling agent, but it appears now that it's a much more remarkable substance than we had first realized. Besides drying out acne, it actually inhibits the growth of *P. acnes* bacteria. There are many forms of benzoyl peroxide, of course. The best are the acetone and water gel formulations and some can be bought over the counter.

Benzoyl peroxides also can dry the skin sufficiently so that it looks as though very little oil is being secreted. Sometimes it's necessary to use a 10 percent or even a 20 percent specially made benzoyl peroxide for this purpose. Benzoyl peroxide can irritate the skin too, so be sure to ask your doctor which strength is right for your skin type.

RETIN-A

Retin-A cream is a form of vitamin A acid applied topically. It appears to correct the defect in the oil gland lining that causes plugging of the canal. However, Retin-A can be an irritating substance. I've had some patients complain of redness and excess drying and peeling when they were on it. But many dermatologists, including myself, prescribe Retin-A, especially in whitehead and blackhead acne. If you can tolerate it, it will do the job. Be prepared for a slight worsening of your condition for up to a few weeks on Retin-A, and realize that it may take up to two to twelve weeks to see the maximum effect.

Some concern has recently arisen about the advisability of using Retin-A; this was prompted by a study showing that Retin-A could cause skin cancers in the presence of sunlight. This study was carried out using a very concentrated solution of Retin-A on rats chosen for their special sun sensitivity. Other studies have shown that Retin-A may protect one from skin cancers, so any resolution is far from final. However, there is now a published warning concerning the use of Retin-A in acne patients who are exposed to a lot of sun. Since Retin-A does cause some thinning of the dead protective layer of the skin, patients are advised not to use it when they are going to be in the sunlight for extended periods. And always use a very high SPF sunscreen

ATTACKING THE OIL FACTORIES WITH RETINOIDS: THE NEW VITAMIN A

Oiliness of facial skin has always been a problem. Some people actually secrete so much oil that even after wiping it off they are able to see it visibly reappear within five minutes on the nose.

Until recently there was nothing that would really decrease oil secretion. Most dermatologists felt that it was important to remove it, but there was no way to shut it down from the inside.

However, there has recently been developed a class of drugs known as the retinoids, which holds tremendous promise for acne patients with excess oil secretion problems. While retinoids have been in use in Europe for many years, they have only recently been released by the Food and Drug Administration (FDA) for use in acne in this country.

Retinoids are chemically altered forms of vitamin A and appear to work in several ways. First, they shut down the production of oil in the oil gland and shrink its size. They also decrease inflammation and have some antibacterial effect. But their prime function in acne is to correct the basic defect that causes plugs down inside the oil glands. No one yet knows exactly how this works, but these drugs, when used by trained dermatologists, are extremely effective. For the first time in acne therapy we may be able to use the word "cure" for up to 94 percent of those people with the most severe type of acne, nodulocystic acne. It's this kind that causes most of the scars on youngsters.

Dr. Gary Peck's study at the National Institutes of Health showed dramatic improvement in acne bumps after treatment with a retinoid called 13-cis-retinoid (Accutane). The medicine is taken by mouth once or twice a day; over about five months, the acne process gradually comes to a halt.

Should your physician choose not to use the drug (see why below), there are other things you may do to help an oiliness problem. Among these are the topically applied form of vitamin A called Retin-A. Retin-A appears to have some of the same effects topically of retinoids given internally in the treatment of acne. However, as I've previously mentioned, it can be irritating, and it works best in whitehead and blackhead acne.

Not everyone can take Accutane. It's only for the 5 percent of acne patients who have the chronic cystic, recalcitrant, scarring kind of acne. And there are complications, such as extreme dryness, chapping, headaches, fatigue, lip irritation, eye dryness, joint and muscle aches, and elevation of fats (cholesterol and triglycerides) in the blood. This necessitates frequent lab tests at the start of therapy. The medicine is also very expensive.

Many patients have asked about the effect of taking just plain oral vitamin A supplements to treat acne. This is a very interesting story, which had its genesis years before in the eye of a very famous dermatologist. For years, dermatologists have prescribed vitamin A with very little success. Dr. Al Kligman, noted acne specialist from Pennsylvania, states that vitamin A will have some of the effects of Accutane if given in near-toxic doses. The problem is that one risks side effects of vitamin A even when treating acne with moderate doses. Vitamin A is one of the fat-soluble vitamins, stored in the liver. Caucasians who first went to Alaska and the Arctic region got very sick when they ate polar bear meat if they included in their diet the liver of the bear. It has such incredible concentrations of vitamin A that it is poisonous. Then, why isn't Accutane toxic? Accutane is not stored in the liver, and it is rapidly excreted. But it's extremely important not to take regular vitamin A if your dermatologist is giving you Accutane. They'll occasionally interact, making each one stronger.

Retinoids can cause defective fetuses in rats and humans. It's absolutely mandatory that pregnant women not take it, and that women taking Accutane not get pregnant while taking it or for one month after their next normal period. Pregnancy tests must be done before the first capsule of Accutane is taken and monthly thereafter because of these pregnancy precautions.

The amazing thing about the retinoids is that their salutary effects are not limited to the treatment of acne. There are many diseases of excess scaliness of the skin that they appear to help marvelously, and, amazingly enough, there are retinoid effects that may hold great promise for everyone's future. Among these is their anticancer effect. Retinoids, when given to experimental animals, appear to reverse precancerous changes in epithelial or skinlike body tissues of bladder and breast. In fact, there has been a remarkable inhibition of breast cancer in certain types of rats who get this disease with incredible facility. If this turns out to be the case, many may get retinoids in the future to reverse precancerous changes. Note that FDA approval for Accutane is only for its use in severe nodulocystic acne.

Taking Accutane for five months often acts as a functional cure in recalcitrant cystic acne, and this effect persists even after the medicine is stopped. Some kids have to be treated a second time, but most clear progressively and have no further problems. So far I've treated over three thousand severe acne patients with this drug and find it the most effective treatment ever for severe cystic acne. There is no doubt about its effectiveness. In fact, when the drug first was approved in 1982, I started taking photographs of every acne patient that received it. After about three hundred sets of these before-and-after pictures, I gave up taking them unless requested to do so by the patients, because there was no longer any doubt that it worked nearly faultlessly in clearing this incredible problem.

SULFA VERSUS SULFUR

Some patients ask if they will have a problem using some of the sulfur-containing anti-acne preparations, since they are allergic to sulfa. They may very well be confusing the words "sulfa" and "'sulfur." Sulfa is an antibiotic given internally for various infections, though allergic reactions can develop to it. While allergic reactions can also (on rare occasions) develop to sulfur used topically, the two drugs are not related and should not cross-react in any way. The sulfur that you may use on your skin is a drying agent that can indeed cause stinging and itching. But this is usually not an allergic reaction, and decreasing the strength of the medicine, or the frequency of its application, can alleviate this problem altogether.

X-RAY THERAPY

It has been known ever since the turn of the century that X-ray therapy can decrease the size of oil glands and help acne. However, researchers found some twenty to thirty years later that X-ray therapy given for acne can cause problems with growths in the thyroid gland in the neck, especially when the neck was not shielded during the x-ray procedure. So most dermatologists are recommending that any patients who have ever been treated with X-ray for acne have a yearly check of their thyroid with a physical examination and certain laboratory tests so that their internist or endocrinologist can follow their thyroid status carefully.

ZINC

Several years ago reports indicated that zinc therapy in acne resulted in early clearing of acne bumps. So most of us jumped on the early bandwagon and gave our patients moderate to high doses of zinc, and then stood back to observe the quick improvement that had been described. However, we succeeded only in nauseating some of our adolescents. Zinc didn't help acne a bit.

I've noticed that the health food stores are two to three years behind in their recommendations on what they think will cure acne. They are currently recommending zinc, and since they can't follow their "patients" as we do in dermatology, they probably will take a lot longer to notice its nausea-producing side effects.

Acne is not a disease related to vitamin deficiency. (In this country, it's very hard even to find someone who's really vitamin-deficient. Even most junk food these days is crammed full of vitamins so that it's nearly impossible to get short-changed in this regard.) Don't bother pursuing acne therapy with vitamins and trace elements.

ATTITUDE AND ACNE

If your child's acne doesn't improve with treatment, the answer may be in three different areas. First, he or she may not be performing all the treatments required by the dermatologist. Take my patient Ronnie, for instance, who was literally dragged into my office by his mother. She pushed him toward me and said, "Treat his acne!" Ronnie was a surly young high school student who was covered with "zits." He really needed help, but I could see he was not about to accept it. I tried to treat him by giving him a lotion that required him to do very little, but this approach failed. Ronnie was certain that the world owed him a smooth, pimple-free face and that he should not have to work for it.

His mother persisted, and month after month he was brought back for reexamination, but he continued to have more and more severe nodular acne and began to scar in spite of my care.

Then one day Ronnie took a complete turnabout and came in by himself to talk to me. He had found a girl in whom he'd developed a romantic interest, but he was afraid she wouldn't like him if he had a "crater face." Now he wanted help.

The change was remarkable. Over the next few months Ronnie began using his topical treatments and taking his capsules, and he continued to improve, with very few permanent scars. After one year he was well stabilized, and his skin looked beautiful. I then began decreasing his medications until he was discharged. Today he's in college with a clear face. I still see him from time to time to treat other minor skin problems, and he never fails to thank me.

Motivation is needed on both sides of the treatment program. In short, the rapport between the physician and the patient is more important in acne than it is in almost any other skin disease. The disease moves rapidly in many patients, leaving its tracks for all to see. It's absolutely crucial that a child have a good working relationship with the dermatologist. If not, it's time to move on to another dermatologist.

Dr. Marsh, my mentor in dermatology, once told me, "Joe, if you can't learn to love treating acne, don't ever get into dermatology. Clearing a kid's acne is a real thrill for me. It'll do the same for you if you learn to treat it and love treating it!" He was right.

If you feel uncomfortable for any reason with a treatment or the rate at which a condition improves, you should discuss it with the dermatologist. Only this can help to clarify any questions.

DIET AND ACNE

Diet is of much less importance than we used to think in acne care. The majority of dermatologists today recommend a well-balanced diet but no definite dietary restrictions. Many of us, however, myself included, recommend avoidance of dairy products, including milk, cheese, and ice cream, and of pork, including bacon and sausage. There must be an agent in these products that encourages acne to form, because patients do better when they avoid them. But as far as I'm concerned, my patients can have all the chocolate, Cokes, candy, nuts, Fritos, potato chips, french fries, and hamburgers they want.

Research shows that there is no significant change in acne caused by eating chocolate. In fact, several years ago a major study was done by Dr. Albert M. Kligman, a well-respected dermatologist and researcher. The study, published in the December 15, 1969, *Journal of the American Medical Association,* was performed at the University Hospital in Philadelphia, Pennsylvania.

Dr. Kligman gave 1,200 calories of chocolate each day to one group of sixty-five acne-prone patients and 1,200 calories per day of nonchocolate-containing look-alike and taste-alike bars to a matched group. No one, not even the researcher, knew which kids were getting the real or the fake chocolate. All the kids were watched for new acne bumps.

After many weeks, the researchers discovered that there was no significant difference between the two groups. So it's true; chocolate's not the acne answer.

However, in my own practice, if patients complain that every time they eat a chocolate bar they get new bumps, I tell them quite frankly that they would be fools to continue eating anything they think causes new lesions.

You see, on a microscopic level, it takes over two to three weeks to make an acne bump, so it's impossible to get all those changes overnight after eating a suspected acne inducer. Maybe someday we'll find out that foods may trigger acne, but in order to do so, we'll have to work with a three-week (or more) history of what was eaten. And that's so difficult that the long-term studies have never been done, except for chocolate.

EMOTIONS— CAN THEY "SCARE UP" ACNE?

As a general rule, I would say that emotions do not have much to do with acne development. The disease is one of plugged oil glands, and no one has yet determined how emotional factors could have a relationship there.

However, in practice, I find that acne often worsens around exam times and other times of severe stress. We are still not sure if this results from the actual stress having a physiological effect on the acne or whether a person just thinks about the acne more during stressful times, possibly pressing or picking at the bumps with greater frequency, or generally ignoring total skin care because of the stress.

REMEMBERING YOUR TREATMENT ROUTINE

Antibiotics have assumed a major role in the treatment of acne, and many of my questions from new acne patients involve the use of antibiotics. One of the most frequent questions concerns the difficulty in remembering to take antibiotics and perform the other elements of a good acne regimen. Remembering to take pills is difficult, for sure. Try to tie the taking of your medicine with some other action repeated in your daily routine. For one of my patients, I recommended he store the tablet bottle in his slipper near his bed at night and keep a glass of water on his nightstand. When he awakened each morning, his foot struck the bottle as he put his slippers on, causing him to remember to take his pill. It worked like a charm! Of course, you could not use this trick if you had small children at home or pets who could reach your medicines. Naturally, all medicines must be kept out of their reach.

If you're on a medicine that may be taken close to meals, I often advise attaching one's toothbrush to the medicine bottle with a rubber band. Then, each time you brush, you'll be reminded about your medicine. This is, of course, contingent upon brushing your teeth after eating!

Tetracycline should be taken on an empty stomach as much as possible. Most forms of tetracycline are greatly affected by meals, especially by the calcium in food. That's generally why milk is to be avoided during acne therapy. But it's even more important that the directions for taking one's medicine be clearly written and clearly understood. A patient of mine named Teresa adequately illustrates this point. Teresa came in with small papular acne, that is, mostly small red bumps. This is usually the easiest type of acne to clear, and it usually clears beautifully on tetracycline capsules. Teresa was instructed to take one capsule three times a day, and on her prescription I wrote "one hour a. c. or two hours p.c." This means "one hour before meals or two hours after meals." Teresa was using her topical medicines faithfully and was taking her capsules, three a day, but was not clearing. Her bumps kept getting worse instead of better even when I increased the dose of tetracycline to four a day.

On her third visit, we were both fairly disturbed with the continual outbreak of new spots, and Teresa asked me if there were any special way to take the medicine. I asked, "Aren't you taking it one hour before meals or two hours after, as I suggested?"

"Did you say, 'before or after meals'?" she asked.

"Yes, as I had written on the prescription," I said, rather impatiently.

"But my bottle says nothing about the time I'm supposed to take it!"

"Do you have it with you?" I asked.

Her hand dipped into her purse and emerged with the bottle. The label read, "Take one capsule three times a day."

"Is that all they had to say about when you should take it?" I asked.

"Yes," she said, "so I've been taking it with meals!"

Now we had the answer to Teresa's antibiotic dilemma. When I instructed her to take it on an empty stomach, she started to clear rapidly.

The exception to this empty stomach rule is a drug called minocycline, a very effective tetracycline derivative, which you need not *necessarily* take on an empty stomach. One problem with minocycline, however, is that it's much more expensive than regular tetracycline. In fact, we usually reserve it for difficult cases of acne because of its cost. However, in cases where patients cannot get themselves to take tetracycline on an empty stomach, it is very easy to take minocycline because they can pop a capsule at mealtime.

The prohibition against food with regular tetracycline has caused some occasional problems. Jennifer, a thirteen-year-old with acne, called me in a panic in the middle of the night stating that she just knew that she was going to die because of the tetracycline she took! "Had she overdosed?" I wondered. Tearful, she said that she had accidentally taken her tetracycline with food and the label specifically said never to do this. She was afraid she would have some terrible reaction. I reassured her that taking the medicine with food just slowed down its absorption and did not cause any toxic effects. Jennifer returned to bed much calmer than when she had called.

If you're on regular tetracycline, you might remember the bottle-in-the-slipper trick mentioned before (provided you don't have any little kids around the house). Also, taking it at nighttime before bed usually provides you with a fairly empty stomach (unless you're a midnight snacker).

The question many patients have is about the duration of antibiotic therapy. They worry about taking a medicine for a long time because of other side effects. This is very important because of the scare implanted in lay persons during the early days of antibiotic therapy. At that time, lay audiences were told that use of antibiotics for a long term would cause a "resistance" to them that would preclude their use in infections at a later date. Actually the group of antibiotics used most often in acne, that is, the tetracyclines, are found to be some of the safest drugs ever invented. While there are side effects, these are uncommon in actual practice.

SIDE EFFECTS OF TETRACYCLINE

The chief side effect, usually occurring in women on doses of 500 to 1,000 milligrams and more per day, is vaginitis. Regular vaginal bacteria are knocked out by the antibiotic and yeasts overgrow. Then an itchy discharge can develop that is quite annoying, but this does not always mean that the patient has to stop the medication. In many cases, since the face is the "window with which one greets the world," it is absolutely necessary to keep up the antibiotic, and in these cases, we usually prescribe vaginal anti-yeast tablets (such as Gyne Lotrimin Tablets, now available over the counter) once or twice a week to prevent yeast infection. There are many other drugs that can perform this function, and your doctor may have another preference. But don't give up hope just because you get an episode of vaginitis. It's a problem that can be very adequately controlled.

Various other side effects of taking tetracycline include nausea and, with minocycline, occasional dizzy spells. Your own dermatologist can brief you on other problems associated with tetracycline in the treatment of acne.

ANTIBIOTICS AND "THE PILL"

Recent reports indicate that tetracycline occasionally diminishes the contraceptive effect of the low-dose birth control pill. Therefore, if you are on the pill, ask your physician whether you should be on tetracycline simultaneously. If your physician doesn't want you on the two together, he or she may want to ask your dermatologist to switch you to erythromycin, which has much the same type of activity that tetracycline has in acne, but which is only about one half to two thirds as effective when given internally. One advantage is that erythromycin usually does not cause vaginitis. If you choose to stay on tetracycline during your acne therapy, you should consider using a second form of contraception.

THE EFFECT OF THE PILL ON ACNE

Oral contraceptives are combinations of estrogens and progestins. While the estrogen component is not acne-causing, the progestin in most pills is broken down by the body into a substance that has androgenic (male hormone) effects. This makes acne worse.

There are, however, several types of birth control pills (BCPs) that are not usually thought to make acne worse. In these BCPs, the progestin is metabolized to an estrogenic substance which may actually help clear acne.

Ask your physician which of these so-called estrogen-dominant types is preferred for you. Your doctor will usually be glad to change types if you haven't had any pill-related problems. For most BCPs, the pill + skin = acne. Ask your doctor for one that will not satisfy this equation.

ANTIBIOTICS AND TEETH

There has been widespread concern over the possibility of tooth staining while a person is taking tetracycline for acne. This is another one of the really misplaced bits of information that gets planted in the lay literature without adequate explanation. Mothers, fathers, and adolescent patients ask this question repeatedly. Tetracycline can cause tooth staining, and even malformation of the teeth, if it's taken before the age of eight. This can also happen to the fetus of a woman who is pregnant, if she takes tetracycline. Therefore, physicians who prescribe tetracycline are very cautious not to give it to young children or pregnant mothers. If neither of these conditions applies, that is, if you're not under the age of eight, and if you're not pregnant, there can be no dental problems with regular tetracycline. With the more potent minocycline, there have been very rare reports of *adult* tooth staining that appears irreversible, so if you are on minocycline for a prolonged time, you should ask your dentist to color-match your teeth so that any color changes may be noticed early and the medicine stopped.

The general recommendation in regard to minocycline would change somewhat in light of this newest information. I'll still treat severe acne patients with the drug, but I'll warn them about the tooth-staining properties of the medicine, and stop it at the first sign of darkening of the enamel of the teeth.

A recent study concerning tetracycline was reviewed at the American Academy of Dermatology meeting in December 1981. A large group of patients on tetracycline for acne were followed carefully over several years, and no problems arose in the adolescents' health, either by physical examination or by lab studies. Of course, as with any prescription medicine, your dermatologist will want to see adolescent patients from time to time, to make sure they are on the right dose of the medication and that all their topical medications are being used correctly.

LEAVE ACNE BUMPS ALONE!

A patient should never operate on his or her own cysts! Squeezing, mashing, or needling these cysts can not only cause a severe infection (when infection may not have been present originally), but it can increase scarring by injecting the rotting cyst material into the surrounding skin.

And, needless to say, using a needle on cysts is to be avoided at all costs. Metal objects can transmit severe infections and even hepatitis. Never approach your face with the intention of doing your own "acne surgery."

HEALING TIME

In these days of air travel, almost everyone has heard of the time delay, called jet lag, in which the body does not adjust quickly enough as one moves from time zone to time zone. The same thing can happen in acne therapy. Some of us have dubbed this time delay between the onset of treatment and the onset of improvement as "zit lag." It's during this period that the skin is adapting to the medicines your dermatologist has prescribed; it can take some two to six weeks before you begin to show an improvement. This is especially true with such agents as topical vitamin A acid and topical antibiotics that have a built-in waiting period before their therapeutic action begins. If you're still not improving nicely four to six weeks down the road, discuss modifications or changes in your acne treatment program with your doctor.

MENSTRUAL OUTBREAKS

Often, period-related acne is well controlled by increasing the amount of internal medicine your physician has prescribed about five to seven days before periods. This should be done only on your dermatologist's advice, however, because some medicines cannot be adjusted this way.

ACNE FOREWARNS MENARCHE

Sometimes we hear the remark that girls as young as nine years old are getting some early acne bumps, even before menstrual periods (menarche) begin. This is very common. Acne often heralds the onset of menstrual periods by as much as two years in children.

FACIAL-CLEANSING ADVICE

Acne is only helped minimally by facial cleansing. It is not dirt that is responsible for acne; it's a problem deep down in the oil glands. So washing frequently helps only insofar as it removes dead skin cells and surface oil. Washing too vigorously or too frequently can even cause new acne, a problem now dubbed "acne mechanica." Washing with the correct anti-acne soaps, however, can result in some drying of the skin and opening up of oil gland openings, which can be beneficial, but just don't overdo it, or expect washing alone to solve your acne problem.

SOAPS

Many different soaps are used in treating the oily skin that usually accompanies acne. Regular glycerine soap is really quite mild. In many of my cases of severe acne, it's much too mild. And for some people it's been found to be frankly comedogenic (whitehead-causing). For my patients, I like mild drying soaps containing sulfur or benzoyl peroxide. I think a mild general drying soap tends to dehydrate the oil gland opening, temporarily enlarging it, allowing normal passage of oil to occur. That's why many of the medications that dermatologists recommend do cause surface drying. One popular manufacturer (Neutrogena) does make a great glycerine acne soap in bar and liquid pump forms, and I find that these special formulations work quite well.

Is Acne Contagious?

Absolutely not. There is no contagious form of acne. Some people interpret genetic passage of the tendency to form acne bumps as a type of contagion, but it is not. However, if both your parents had severe acne and you do, too, this bears out the generally accepted theory that if each of your parents had bad acne you have about an 80 percent chance of having it also.

Other Factors in Acne Care

Changing pillowcases and towels will not aid in the resolution of acne. Again, this old saw that acne is due to dirt is completely untrue. However, the sulfur medications sometimes used at night tend to flake off on the pillow and it may be necessary for that reason to change pillowcases.

Nose "Blackheads and Whiteheads"

The nose is a characteristic place for blackheads to occur, but most children do not have true blackheads. Most of them have simple dots at the top of columns of oil that lead down into the oil glands on the nose. These are usually quite deep but are not the massively obstructed oil glands represented in blackheads. It's often possible to squeeze the nasal skin gently and coax these tiny dots to the surface where they can be wiped off. Certainly you should not be doing your own acne surgery, but this can show you the type of lesion or spot that these are.

    Treatment is very difficult. The black dot is not dirt, but a pigment called melanin picked up from the surrounding skin cells. All the washing in the world will help this only slightly. Agents such as the potent forms of benzoyl peroxide, which I've already mentioned, can help lighten these lesions chronically. However, the tiny dots (even in the middle-aged patient) are usually not visible at a conversational distance, so the sufferer need not feel too self-conscious about them.

THE SUN AND ACNE

Sunlight usually helps acne, but reports over the last several years indicate that intense sunlight or sunlamp exposure can actually induce new bumps. This is becoming more and more a problem because of the desire of adolescents for a dark suntan. Some of these kids come in with a tremendous crop of acne lesions just because of excess sun exposure.

Keep in mind that the sun actually damages the skin. This damage consists not only of wrinkles but of the induction of pre-malignant spots and actual malignant skin cancers. Most dermatologists do not prescribe sunlight for the treatment of acne. The major exception is in widespread acne of the back and trunk in which phototherapy is sometimes used as an adjunct in treatment.

My mentor in dermatology, Dr. Glenn Marsh, is very fond of telling a story about one patient, a young woman named Stacy, who showed up in his office with the most incredible case of acne that he had ever seen. Stacy had terrible nodulocystic and bleeding lesions on the nape of her neck, all over her face, the front of her neck, and the chest and back all the way to the beltline. In short, she was a total mess!

"What in the world happened to you?" the dermatologist said.

"Not much, just a little sun bathing," she replied.

"Did you put anything on your skin?"

"Well, I found this new preparation my friend had recommended, which gave me a fantastic rapid tan," she replied.

"Well, what was it?" he asked, "Essence of Acne?"

"Nope. Sheer, fresh, 10-W-30 motor oil!" she exclaimed.

He had no problem figuring out that it wasn't entirely the sun that had caused her acne. Motor oil on the skin of a human being can cause acne almost anywhere!

SHOTS FOR ACNE

Some patients develop huge knots on the face that are actually acne cysts. They are spots of tremendous inflammation that can be decreased by injecting medicine right into them.

The medicine used is a type of cortisone, usually one called triamcinolone. Triamcinolone in small quantities inside the cyst can make it shrink until the body's natural defenses reabsorb the cystic sac. You should certainly discuss these injections with your doctor as they are usually very desirable in order to decrease the healing time of these scarring lesions.

You should know, however, that there is a risk of atrophy in the area below the cyst injected with this material. This means that in some cases the fat layer beneath the cyst is caused to thin out at least temporarily. This can leave a small sunken spot for a few weeks. This is why most of us choose to use a very low-strength medicine that may have to be repeatedly injected every three to four weeks. Usually this low-strength dilution of triamcinolone will not cause the fat atrophy.

Ordinary acne bumps have no cavity within them to speak of so that there is no room to put the steroid material. Any attempt to inject a small papule or bump usually results in leakage of the medicine out into the surrounding skin, causing more problems with sunken spots.

RESTORING ACNE-SCARRED SKIN

You now know a lot about what causes acne and about what can be done when it develops. But what if you found this book too late? What if your cystic acne occurred before we had Accutane and powerful antibiotics? Take a look around and you'll see dozens of ex-acne sufferers for whom our dermatological miracles came too late. Does that mean it's too late to help your scarring? Absolutely not!

There are several methods developed in the last few years from which you and your doctor can choose to resurface your scars. Usually a combination of dermatological and plastic-surgical techniques are used. Many dermatologists and dermatologic surgeons can perform the whole restoration process, so asking your doctor is the only way. Not all techniques will work for everybody, and it's important that you know what you're in for.

Take dermabrasion, for example. It's a major procedure fraught with complications, and sometimes a single dermabrasion won't do the whole job. Let's take a closer look.

THE DERMABRASION DILEMMA

Dermabrasion, or facial planing, is used to recontour and smoothe the surface of the skin. It is a procedure that is not to be taken lightly, since it causes a tremendous amount of temporary disability (weeping, pain, crusting, and possible secondary infection) and some long-term disabilities (several months or longer of altered skin color, sun sensitivity, and possible further scarring). In this procedure, the dermatologist or plastic surgeon briefly freezes the skin and then sands off the upper layers with a small diamond-coated wheel or brush. This is done under general or local anesthesia.

The sanding is continued until tiny bleeding points are reached in the skin. This indicates that the proper depth for scar removal has been reached. Depending on the type of scarring you have, one such operation may suffice; if the scars are deep, two operations may be needed. While there are hazards associated with dermabrasion, such as infection, variation in skin color, and even scarring induced by the operation, it is, in general, a safe procedure when done by skilled hands. It is not always possible, of course, to sand out every scar with the first procedure or even with the second one. You should be sure to discuss all the pros and cons of this treatment with your dermatologist or plastic surgeon.

Very frequently dermabrasions are done in the offices of dermatologists and plastic surgeons. This can avoid the high cost of hospitalization, but the procedure itself is fairly expensive, ranging from $1,000 to $2,500, depending on the surgeon and on the size of the area that must be abraded. Most dermabrasions are full face, because if there is any pigment or texture change in the skin, it's more desirable to have the entire face look the same.

If the dermabrasion is done to treat active acne (as is sometimes the case) most insurance policies will reimburse the patient. However, even if the policy does not reimburse, dermabrasion, like other cosmetic procedures, can function as a tax deduction. Talk to your physician and your tax adviser and health insurance company concerning this *before* you make plans.

Nothing can restore the skin to its "pre-acne" quality. But dermabrasion, sometimes combined with chemical peels and other rehabilitative efforts, which we will discuss, can result in a better appearance.

If you have significant wrinkling due to age and sun changes, a combined procedure of a facelift and dermabrasion may help you to a greater degree. Often the lax skin of a patient in his or her late forties or fifties who has had severe acne as a kid can be radically smoothed by a facelift, even when *not* combined with a dermabrasion.

Dermabrasion should not be regarded as a cure-all for scarring or any other problem. There are complications with the procedure, and everyone who undergoes it should be fully aware of these complications. Be sure you fully inquire about complications before you undergo any surgical procedure.

COLLAGEN IMPLANTS

Advances in scar therapy include the development of Zyderm for injection into scars caused by acne and other conditions. This material is a thick gel produced by chemically breaking up leather into its component parts. The process makes it very similar to human collagen, the support network for the skin. That's the part of the skin that actually holds it together, just like the leather in a leather coat.

Zyderm was tested with thousands of patients for several years prior to its approval by the FDA and its release in the spring of 1981.

The substance of collagen can be equated to a group of small molecular bricks that cement themselves together under the skin when the correct body temperature and environment are reached.

Zyderm should be used only by dermatologists specially trained by the Collagen Corporation. Some—not all—acne scars respond beautifully to it. The material is injected below saucerlike, gently rolling acne scars, and elevates the center of the scar, thus making shadowing in the scar a lot less noticeable. The scars do not actually go away but their visibility is in most instances greatly reduced.

Treatment with Zyderm for acne scars or any other scars consists of two steps. The first is a test injection: a small amount is injected under the skin of the forearm and allowed to sit in place for a month to detect any possible allergies. If, after a month, the dermatologist finds no sign of redness or firmness, which might indicate allergy, then a second test injection is usually done up near the forehead hairline. Then, two weeks later (assuming a negative test), the injections of the scars can begin.

There are, however, several groups of patients who cannot be injected with Zyderm. These are patients who have autoimmune diseases, a type of allergic reaction to one or more of the body's own organs. Chief among these is rheumatoid arthritis. Others include Crohn's disease, Graves' disease, discoid lupus, systemic lupus, Sjogren's syndrome, ulcerative colitis, Reiter's syndrome, psoriatic arthritis, progressive systemic sclerosis, polymyositis, and polyarteritis.

COLLAGEN INJECTION

While the specific number of treatments is determined by the results after the first injection, it is possible to say in general that most acne patients need at least three and sometimes four or five injections to maximally correct scars. After the one-month waiting period to determine if the skin test is negative, injections can be performed every two weeks until the therapy is completed.

Multiple scars are usually treated in a single session. Often, I do an entire side of the face in an acne-scarred patient and sometimes the entire facial surface. There is no limit to the number of lesions that can be treated in each session, but, practically speaking, one or two milliliters of material is the usual dose injected at one sitting if indeed the patient has that many scars to warrant usage of that much material.

Since Zyderm is injected into the skin, there is no reason to suspect that subsequent skin peelings or dermabrasions would affect the treatments in any way. Many dermatologists and plastic surgeons combine procedures.

How long lasting is the Zyderm material? Based on collagen replacement studies, there is no reason to suspect that it may not be present for six months to eight months after the initial injection. In fact, some patients return just for a yearly touch-up with the medicine. The medicine works best for the types of multiple rolling scars we see after cystic acne, but not as well in the tiny punctate-, sharply demarcated-, ice-pick-type scars we see in some kids who have had scarring acne.

COMPLICATIONS OF COLLAGEN

The main complication, of course, as I have previously mentioned, is allergy to the medicine. While a test injection usually filters out those who are allergic to the medicine, there have been several reports of facial reaction even after negative skin testing. This involved tender bumps lasting several months. Keep in touch with your skin therapist if you have any problems whatsoever with your injections.

Other possible complications include (rarely) infection and sun sensitivity in the injection sites. Sun sensitivity causes temporary redness. This can also occasionally occur if a patient drinks alcohol after having the injections. In general, it is wise for Zyderm-injected patients to get minimal sun and avoid alcohol for several days after the injections.

In summary, Zyderm collagen implants have become one of the most useful tools in the dermatologist's arsenal for restoring scarring skin to its normal look. Realize, however, that it does not solve scarring once and for all. It just alters the contour of the skin so that the scarring that is present is less obvious.

In this regard, I remember Maria, a patient who had a special type of acne the French call *"acne excoriée des jeunes filles."* This means severely picked-at acne of young women. Maria had a tremendously disturbing youth, and as an expression of this discontent she began picking at the few acne lesions she developed as a teenager.

She became so embroiled with her physical appearance that she would actually try to dig out any small imperfection, such as an acne bump, with her fingernail. The result: large scarred craters in place of acne bumps. When she came to see me her scars were a quarter of an inch deep, and she had become a virtual recluse.

After a negative skin test, we began a program of biweekly Zyderm collagen implant injections that rapidly filled her craters to the point where shadowing from overhead lights was minimal. The craters themselves would never go away, and the pigment she had scratched out probably would never return, but with minor cosmetic adjustments she was able to restore her social functioning to a more normal basis. Now she writes me every few months to let me know how well she is doing with her "new life." It's frankly as close to a cosmetic miracle as I have ever seen!

PUNCH EXCISION OF SCARS

Chicken-pox-type scars or acne scars which resemble them have a fairly sharp edge that makes the elevation of them quite difficult. Often these are best treated by plastic surgical intervention with dermabrasion ("skin sanding") or actual excision, or cutting out of the scar.

Some skin surgeons prefer to cut out the scar with a small punch biopsy, or cookie-cutterlike instrument, exactly the same size as the scar itself. Then this tiny punched-out piece of skin pops up to skin level, where it is sewn in place. Later, if there is any irregularity to the skin, a local dermabrasion can be done to smooth it out. This technique is very effective in making these spots look better.

BACK SCARS

Unfortunately, back scars are the hardest to treat. This is the case where the old cliché, "an ounce of prevention is worth a pound of cure," actually does apply. The scars on the back are so extensive in some kids that almost no therapy helps. I find that the woven, unmedicated acne cleansing pads (like the Buf Puf) used with slightly drying soaps containing sulfur or benzoyl peroxide work best to smooth out some small scars, but we really can do practically nothing at this time to help the big sunken scars on the back. Theoretically, Zyderm would work, but small mountains of it might be needed to show significant effect.

You may have noticed from time to time that some acne lesions on the back heal with a nodule or bump above the surface. These are usually reddish at first. They are solid, almost rockhard. These are called hypertrophic scars and are extremely difficult to treat. Sometimes the peeling slush treatment with carbon dioxide, made up by mixing acetone with crushed dry ice, or a spray-freezing treatment with liquid nitrogen does help in combination with injections of cortisone right into the scars. Various types of cortisone are used for these shots. (Note: These treatments are to be administered only by your doctor; they are never to be attempted by the patient!)

It's these terrifically damaging scars that we hope the new retinoid drugs will help avert in the future.

ACNE IN OLDER PERSONS

Acne is not necessarily a disease of the young. Sometimes it lasts into the forties, which can be quite disturbing to the patient and his or her family. Lumps on the face of a person in the forties require a different approach to diagnosis and to treatment. These lumps are either acne or a condition called rosacea (pronounced *rose ASH uh*). More about rosacea later. We're seeing more and more cases of acne (even the more severe nodulocystic kind that some older patients appear to have) in people well beyond their teenage years. Although we think a lot of this has to do with the use of cosmetics by women, we suspect that acne persists in men because of the constant presence of large amounts of male hormone in a person who has a genetic heritage for a predisposition to acne.

WHITEHEADS IN THE ELDERLY

Whiteheads and blackheads on the faces of the elderly are often a problem known as Favre-Racachout syndrome, also known as nodular elastoidosis with cysts and comedones. Sounds complicated, but it really does describe it well. The problem results from the loose skin (elastoidosis) that accompanies TMB (too many birthdays) and damage from years of sunlight exposure. Small blackheads (comedones) form all over the upper cheeks and eye areas (the orbits), which need a type of acne surgery (expression of blackheads by the dermatologist).

A face-lift usually helps the Favre-Racachout problem too. At least 60 percent of my patients with this problem have the loose eyelid skin that is just ripe for what the plastic surgeons call a blepharoplasty, or lid job. This is one of the neatest operations ever invented, and it can make you look years younger. Think about it!

Treatment of this blackhead condition centers around pushing out the whiteheads and trying to prevent them in the future. We use a little tool something like a hairpin. It's called a comedo (blackhead) extractor. The trick is knowing how to do the procedure so you don't injure yourself. It's for this reason that I wouldn't ask you to go down to the drugstore and buy yourself one of these gadgets. Have an expert, your dermatologist, do it.

By the way, this problem of whiteheads and blackheads around the eyes is one of the all-time most popular "Say, Doc" diseases. That's a condition discovered on a relative of an office patient as the patient leaves the room. Usually the patient leaves first and the relative hangs behind for a mini-office visit, and says, "Say, Doc, what do you suppose these white things are on my cheeks?"

ACNE INDUCED BY PHYSICAL PRESSURE

As we have said, acne can be a process that does not resolve until middle age in some men. While there are not very many sixty-five-year-olds with acne, it's impossible to tell the individual patient when his or her own case of acne will subside. We believe that treatment of acne may keep the patient asymptomatic; that is, the patient may have a tendency for the condition to occur, but this tendency is effectively masked while the disease essentially burns itself out. Treatment, in other words, is a protective screen in front of the acne forest fire, and we keep the screen up as long as necessary to prevent damage. Almost everyone does indeed stop forming new bumps as they age.

Sometimes there are causes you would not normally suspect for acne in certain regions of the body, for instance, the back. I treated a salesman with back acne who had no lesions whatsoever on his face. But he drove about 500 to 800 miles a week, and he thought that might have something to do with the extensive acne on his back.

Sure enough, when we went out to examine his car, we found it had vinyl seat covers. He found that after sitting on this occlusive surface for some time, his back was very hot and sweaty. When I started him on a treatment regimen, I also advised him to get a soft sheepskin cover for his seat. This resulted in a prompt resolution of his back acne. The salesman had developed what is known as tropical acne—acne that results from intense heat and occlusion of the skin, combined with the bad influence of widespread pressure upon skin that bears oil glands. This results in tremendous and explosive acne in some persons!

The most striking case I have ever seen of pressure-induced acne was in a young woman named Sherry who had very severe acne on the right cheek only. The bumps were so close together that her whole cheek was covered with papular, or small-bump, acne.

I asked her if she leaned her face on her hand. Sherry said she was very careful not to do this because she thought that might have something to do with her condition.

I put Sherry on a treatment program, but she didn't do very well. The explosive acne continued to develop in exactly the same area. One day her husband came in with her when I was asking her about local influences on the skin.

I asked her again if something were pressing on the skin of the right side of her face. Her husband then blurted out the fact that she slept on her right hand every single night.

Now it was clear that Sherry's hand was causing her acne. So I prescribed a soft, brown garden glove for her to wear only at night and asked her to try to keep her pillow between her hand and her face. Sherry's acne cleared almost magically. Since then I've been quite impressed with the effect of pressure on the skin in causing acne.

Helmet and chin-strap acne are two variants that really annoy some sports-loving teens. Sometimes it is extraordinarily difficult to get these areas cleared without stopping the pressure by the strap. Drying agents used on the forehead and chin during football season can help calm the eruption, but for the most part, it's necessary to alleviate the pressure. This can be done by padding the chin-strap area and helmet contact points with a very soft felt material. It's not perfect, but it may help.

DERMATOPATHIC LYMPHADENOPATHY

Occasionally victims of severe acne notice swellings in the neck areas below and underlying their complexion problems. This condition is called dermatopathic lymphadenopathy. This means that the tiny lymph glands under the chin area are draining the products of inflammation from your acne areas. These products lodge temporarily within the glands, irritate them, and cause them to swell. The lumps can get quite tender and sometimes persist until the acne itself has come under control. The presence of inflammation in the lymph glands of the neck will often lead your dermatologist to consider that there may be strep or staph infection down inside the facial acne bumps. For this reason, your doctor may choose to change your antibiotic to one that will knock out these bacteria. This change would be temporary, just until the supervening infection is wiped out, and then you would most probably be put back on your routine anti-acne antibiotics.

COSMETICS AND ACNE

As I've said before, acne is a disease of an ever older age group these days, a fact that has distressed many of us in dermatology.

We believe there are two general reasons for this. First, we have tried over the years to increase patient awareness of what can be done for acne so that many men and women now consult dermatologists earlier for a few bumps rather than put up with them until they scar and go away on their own. It's this patient concern that has brought about the demand for ever more effective acne medications.

Second, cosmetic industry leaders, while doing what they can to protect against cosmetic-induced acne, have not completely succeeded. That is, many cosmetics are still inducing acne. This situation is compounded for older women since our looks-conscious society demands a continued youthful appearance. The result often is an increasing use of cosmetics to mask minor flaws. Then the cosmetics themselves can cause a plugging of oil glands, or some change in the secretion of oil, which we see later as "acne cosmetica" (acne induced and sustained by cosmetics).

Acne cosmetica is a very severe and widespread problem. It was discovered when researchers were testing the inner ears of rabbits for the irritant potential of cosmetics. Some of their results were not irritation, but whiteheads and blackheads on the rabbit ear skin. So substances such as cold creams and makeup are now used as the *test substances* to produce experimental acne in which new therapeutic medications may be tried!

Now I'm not trying to kill off the cosmetic industry. I think cosmetics are a prime requisite in our society today, and I would not ask women to go without them, since there are now systems that can be used which do not induce new acne. Some of the best systems of cosmetics that do not generally cause acne are Allercreme, Lancome, and Clinique brands. However, even within these brand groupings I would advise avoidance of the companies' "acne treatment programs," because they are generally not effective and can result in delay of treatment of your acne when what you may need most is to see the dermatologist as soon as possible.

Until these newer, noncomedogenic cosmetic systems came along, my standard axiom was "A little makeup, a little paint, sure makes acne where it ain't!" So if you have any tendency toward acne, and if you want to give yourself a fighting chance, you should use one of the brands recommended here or ask your dermatologist for one that is preferred by him or her. Research shows that to do otherwise may be gambling with the only face you've got.

HORMONES—
THE MATCH THAT LIGHTS THE ACNE FIRE

Often, women who have undergone "surgical menopause" notice a drastic increase in the number and severity of acne bumps on their faces. If the surgeons removed the ovaries, which would result in a drastic drop in the amount of estrogen in the system (ovaries make estrogen), it is likely that acne will worsen if a person has a tendency toward it. Estrogen, as you know, is a female hormone that can combat acne. Therefore, if ovaries were removed, there is a sudden decrease in the amount of estrogen in the system. This allows the small amount of male hormones (androgens) to stimulate oil glands and cause new acne. We often see this happen, albeit somewhat more slowly, around the time of natural menopause, when a few bumps come on very gradually.

There are some diseases that manifest themselves first by a low-grade case of acne. Some of these diseases are endocrine in nature and involve such problems as ovarian cysts or pituitary or even adrenal difficulties. If your doctor did not remove your ovaries when your uterus was removed and your acne persists, have your doctor check you for endocrine gland problems.

The treatment of acne in an older age group is basically the same as the treatment in teenagers except that such patients will not need as much drying in order to clear. Often antibiotics are necessary to suppress the outbreak of new lesions. That's where the drug tetracycline comes in handy. It can slow down or stop the appearance of new bumps by preventing the rotting of oil in the sebaceous glands within the skin.

EXPENSE OF ACNE CARE

Unfortunately, acne care tends to be moderately expensive. And the age-old adage that you get what you pay for may certainly apply in acne therapy, since some of the medicines used are quite expensive. But they are also effective. You might ask your dermatologist for samples of medications to cut down on costs. Many dermatologists supply their patients with samples, and it certainly never hurts to ask.

We sometimes hear a patient say that they would have come in earlier for acne treatment, but that their insurance plan would not cover "acne and other cosmetic conditions." When we dermatologists hear such statements we go ballistic! Acne *IS* an illness, just as much as diabetes or heart failure is. It is a painful disease that may cause scarring and emotional problems for life. In this regard it deserves to be covered by *any* insurance plan that treats those other more "conventional" diseases, that's for sure. We often write letters to such companies informing them of patients' plights and the potential and real problems involved with their physical health and acne. As yet, as long as a patient didn't sign a specific waiver of coverage for acne per se, which I have heard of in certain instances, you should be covered by your major medical or other health insurance plan. And you can show the officials of your plan this book to help convince them!

Allergies

ALLERGIES ARE FOR LIFE!

If you have an allergy to some component, you'll probably never lose it. That type of allergy is mediated, or caused, by certain cells in your body called lymphocytes. This type of white blood cell is especially competent at picking up substances or chemicals from outside the body and recognizing them as "foreign." And, good little police officers that they are, the lymphocytes react against anything recognized in such a way by forming antibodies. They, in turn, cause the red, itchy rash to occur.

Antibodies are the tremendous protective chemicals that keep all of us alive each day by fighting off all sorts of infections, eliminating some microscopic malignancies, and performing a million other functions we never think about.

COSMETIC ALLERGIES

"I've been using the same cosmetics for years!" That statement is the most common remark of patients with cosmetic allergy. It's also the most inaccurate. The skin, magnificent organ that it is, can learn how to become allergic to a substance even after years of using it without problems. In dermatology, we see this happen constantly.

A patient named Meri sought my help with a chronically swollen eyelid. She had used the same cosmetics for many years, and had had this facial reaction for only a month. As a busy young executive, she had not had the time to get the problem checked out earlier.

When we patch-tested her to the standard American Academy of Dermatology (AAD) kit of allergens, she showed a strong positive reaction to formalin, a substance usually used as a preservative. Looking through Meri's cosmetics revealed that her nail polish contained (at that time) formalin.

"I'll bet you're in one heck of a hurry most of the time, right?" I asked.

"Sure, Dr. Bark. I always seem to have ten things on my schedule, and nine of them are overdue."

"Put your nail polish on in a hurry, too?"

"Usually. It's a quick job in the mornings."

"Aha!" I exclaimed. "That's where you're getting the formalin."

"Beg your pardon?"

"You see, Meri," I explained, "when you run out of the house with slightly soft nail polish, you've been touching your lids occasionally. This leaves traces of the very material you're allergic to right on your poor eyelids. And that's what's causing your dermatitis."

"Fantastic!" she said. "But does that mean that I can never again wear my favorite nail polish?"

"No, not at all. All you have to do to make sure you don't react to it is to be absolutely sure that the polish is dry when you are ready to go in the morning. And to make sure of that, all you have to do is the 'dry test.' "

"What's the dry test?" she asked.

"Just touch a cotton ball lightly to the nails when you think they're dry. If any fibers from the cotton are left on the nail, then you'll have to give it more time . Be sure to do this when you have some extra time, so that you can get an idea of how long it takes to really get your polish dry."

Meri's problem disappeared, and she was able to continue using the polish. She also took care to avoid other substances with formalin, such as some shampoos, certain toothpastes, permanent-press fabrics, and so forth.

LIPS AND LIPSTICK RASHES

One of the more frequent complaints heard in the dermatologist's office is one concerning a woman's lips. I had a patient, Marcia, whose lips were red as fire, and this without lipstick! They were raw, cracked, and swollen, even outside the margins of the vermilion area, the area we see as red on the lips. She said that she had been having a problem with dry lips for several months, and that she religiously used her lipstick and moisturizing lip balm, but nothing seemed to help. She wondered, as so many people do, how she could possibly be allergic to a substance or product that she had been using for years.

The answer is simple, but unfortunately incompletely understood. Our bodies recognize some part of the lipstick formula as a foreign substance and react against it. Some women accurately recognize the allergy has occurred and switch lipsticks, hoping to avoid it. What is not often realized is that many lipsticks, and other cosmetics for that matter, have common ingredients, especially the preservatives, which frequently cause allergy.

The real key is to be patch-tested to find out the exact chemical that has caused the allergy. Then you can carefully pick your next lipstick to exclude that chemical.

Important: The ingredients of cosmetics are sometimes changed without notice from the manufacturer. This is another reason you could develop an allergy to a cosmetic you've used for some time.

NICKEL ALLERGIES— A PROBLEM THAT SHOWS YOUR TRUE METTLE

Some women (and occasionally men) have a problem wearing most types of jewelry. They itch around earlobes where they wear pierced earrings, or around their necks when they try to wear good necklaces. These are the classic symptoms of "nickel allergy." This is almost always the problem when a jewelry rash is acquired. Pierced earrings are often the culprit. That's where most women first come into contact with the element nickel, and that's where the lymphocytes first pick it up and recognize it as a foreign substance.

Once again, the real shame is that if you get allergic to nickel, you're apt to be allergic to it for a long, long time. A lab technician named Julie at the Medical College of Georgia developed nickel allergy after getting her ears pierced in a shopping center. Since she had to deal with metals such as nickel in the lab all day, Julie was really in trouble.

Unluckily, she demonstrated a fact about nickel allergy that no one likes to think about. Unlike other allergies that fade rather rapidly once the offending allergen or chemical is removed, Julie's rash hung on for months after a single exposure. Nickel metal binds to the protein in the upper skin layers, and the skin keeps reacting to it, thus causing extended dermatitis.

What could we do for Julie? We tried everything to get her back into wearing her favorite earrings. Some of our methods worked, and others did not.*

Whenever possible, we asked Julie not to wear her earrings. This helped somewhat by limiting her exposure to the offending metal. We coated them with clear nail polish, so that the nickel would not contact her skin so easily, when she absolutely had to wear them.

We treated her with a medicine called Kenalog spray, which leaves a resin behind to coat the ear hole and protect it from the nickel. Kenalog spray also contains a potent cortisone that treats the rash.

We tested all her jewelry items with a chemical test kit available to all dermatologists, called the dimethylglyoxime (DMG) kit, which revealed that several other items were nickel-positive. We eliminated these from her contact as well.

Since all our efforts were only partially successful, we asked a local jeweler to replace Julie's DMG-positive earring posts with ones made of surgical grade stainless steel, the only metal universally safe to wear by those allergic to nickel. It contains nickel, but it's so tightly bound into the alloy that it can't escape to cause dermatitis. That's when we residents discovered a much easier way to get Julie back into earrings and jewelry again. At the American Academy of Dermatology meeting one December, I found a display by a little company in New York that makes very nice, certified nickel-free, hypoallergenic earrings and other jewelry, called Ear-Eze. Their address is:

Ear-Eze H & A Enterprises, Inc.
143-19 25th Avenue
P.O. Box 489
Whitestone, NY 11357

---

*First, of course, we were interested in getting her back to work safely. We had her wear fresh cotton gloves or latex gloves in her work, and change them frequently. This helped greatly.

These folks are very cooperative in supplying nickel-free items directly to patients. Write them, and they send you an order form for their beautiful set of color catalogs.

Since an ounce of prevention is worth a pound of cure, women should take care to ensure that the original piercing of their ears is done with completely nickel-free materials. My dermatology professor used to dread nickel dermatitis so much that when young women would ask him if he'd pierce their ears, he'd say, "Sure, I'll pierce your ears, if you'll let me put a ring in your nose at the same time!" Oddly enough, due to societal changes, that turned out to be true. We are now starting to see reactions of nickel dermatitis around the nose studs that a lot of kids wear these days. Maybe the message is that the body does not like foreign substances no matter how decorative. Kids should at least think about this when they consider piercing-type jewelry of any kind.

While we have come a long way since then, I still insist that completely nickel-free posts be used. And you don't find those very often at department store piercing salons. You may, however, convince them to let you take the piercing posts to your dermatologist so they can be tested for the presence of nickel. It's simple, and should definitely be done first, to make sure your posts are surgical-grade stainless steel. Once you've got nickel dermatitis, it's too late. Most dermatologists have the "DMG Kit" and can test for the presence of nickel in any metal without hurting the item one bit. It's a neat test and can save you or your kid lots of worry, itching, pain, and expense if you do this test *before* you get "pierced."

I wish I could say that "good gold," like fourteen-carat and eighteen-carat items were safe in all circumstances, but unfortunately, quite a bit of fourteen-karat gold contains leachable nickel, that is, nickel that can be drawn out by sweat, water, detergents, and so forth. So to be safe, you should stick to stainless steel.

Some patients want to know how to treat the piercing site after the procedure is done. Isopropyl alcohol (common rubbing alcohol) is really quite a good antibacterial agent. It probably keeps the number of bacteria so low that the probability of an infection of the pierced ear tract is remote. But once the tract made by the piercing instrument is fully healed, such infections are extremely rare anyway. So it's probably wise to use alcohol for the first three weeks or so, until the holes are fully healed.

FOOD FACIALS

People will sometimes believe anything that is in print. And while I realize that *you* are now reading printed words on a subject, some of the nonexpert-supplied information we get is downright incorrect, if not dangerous. This applies to the so-called food cosmetics, in which people were told to put lime juice and vitamin E on the face. Incredible! Lime juice is one of the most potent photosensitizers known. That means that, if you are exposed to even small amounts of sunlight, a fairly violent rash can occur. It's all right to eat limes, but never let the juice or rind come in contact with your skin.

Interestingly, topical vitamin E should be off limits for the skin because of the propensity it has to cause topical skin allergy. We have seen frequent cases of itchy rashes when it is applied to the skin.

Aloe

JUST ANOTHER GIMMICK

There's really no good evidence one way or the other, that the aloe vera (the "burn plant") juice actually does any harm or good. It's been rumored for years that it was good to break open the thick leaves of this plant and apply the juice to minor burns or other injuries. In order to be at all effective, the aloe juice must be in this strength, just as it comes out of the broken plant. It appears that the concentrations of aloe currently available in cosmetics and other topically applied forms are not effective because they are not in a strong enough form.

Angiomas

Many people develop red, discrete bumps on the skin as they age. These tiny reddish bumps are called cherry angiomas (De Morgan's spots). They are another benign sign of TMB (too many birthdays), composed of hundreds of dilated (wide-open) capillaries in the skin surface. They indeed do arise more frequently in families with a history of them, and the chances of your passing these lesions on to your kids is excellent.

Note carefully that these lesions do not ordinarily bleed, unless they have occurred in an area of trauma, such as the shaving areas. But if they are nicked and start to bleed, they're tough to stop. They also slowly enlarge with time. I've seen ones as big as an eraser by the hundreds on patients' chests.

Although from a medical standpoint they really don't need to be treated, patients often want them off for cosmetic reasons. In that case, we zap them with a tiny current from an electric needle. They'll usually go away without a trace after this procedure.

Baby Skin

WHAT TO USE AND NOT TO USE

Each time a newborn baby is delivered, an amazing counting process begins. Every parent wants to make sure that his or her baby came off the assembly line with all its parts. After checking the number of fingers and toes, new parents then begin to inspect that fantastic material covering them, skin. It's an examination process that will proceed for the rest of the child's life.

Isn't it incredible that in just nine short months the embryonic skin develops every one of the thousands of structures within it that are present in adult skin: oil glands, hair, hair muscles, nerves, blood vessels, sweat glands—everything! And it all works. A newborn's skin is already such a fantastic air-conditioning unit that babies can easily grow cold because of its efficient heat transfer. In fact, that's why babies wear stocking caps—their head skin comprises a much greater proportion of their total body skin than does the head skin of an adult.

Most of us manage our own skins pretty well, but we panic when it comes time to tend the delicate skin of the newborn. The difference is that we're not struggling to survive in a totally new, completely alien atmosphere, replete with threats of yeast in diapers, irritation from soaps and lotions, and a thousand other threats every day.

DIAPER RASH

It's always been amazing how little is understood by the general medical community (let alone parents) about what causes diaper rash. The diaper dilemma was solved for me by a few simple words from one of the most respected pediatricians ever known, the late Dr. Warren Wheeler of the University of Kentucky. While I was doing an admission physical exam on a baby one day, Dr. Wheeler noticed that my patient's groin was as red as a fire truck. He ambled over to the baby's bed with his quick little hopping step, put his hands on his hips, and peered at my patient with his big bespectacled eyes as I went through the physical exam (quite nervously, under the gaze of the department chairman). Finally he blurted out excitedly, "Doctor, why do you think that little peanut has that diaper rash?"

"Well, judging by my lecture notes, I'd say that it's probably ammonia, Dr. Wheeler."

"No, I mean why does he have a *diaper* rash? My point, Dr. Bark, is that this little pumpkin probably has a diaper rash because he's wearing a diaper. Leave that diaper off, and you'll cure him, sure as shootin'!" He walked off briskly, smiling to himself that he had given yet another med student a tip that would serve him a lifetime.

That very simple fact, which should be obvious to every physician, mother, and father concerned with diaper rash, often completely escapes their minds. Since those days in medical school, I've successfully treated hundreds of cases of diaper rash just by having the parents keep the child out of diapers whenever possible.

Just as important, however, since most parents will not avoid diapers altogether because of the mess involved, is the use of the right type of diaper. Our modern, disposable, throwaway age has led us to believe that disposable diapers are the final answer to baby care. The simple and unavoidable truth of infancy is "what eats, excretes," and the problem of diaper rash is avoidable with the proper "care and maintenance" of your kid's south side.

This means using the old-fashioned cotton diapers instead of the disposable type. Yes, I know this book is slamming shut all across the nation, but for any kid who has a tendency toward diaper dermatitis, this tip is crucial to prevention. Let me explain further about the reasoning behind the use of cloth diapers. For years we have been looking after the convenience and ease of the parents at the expense of the babies who have to wear disposable diapers. The problem grew even worse when the plastic covering was invented for the paper diaper. The plastic keeps the parent away from the wetness, not the child!

We'd all like to think that every mother changes her baby's diapers as soon as they are wet, but in practice we know the system is less than perfect, and the baby often does sit in urine for some time before changing, even in the most meticulous of families. The crucial question is, who sits in the wet urine? You guessed it! It's the baby in that disposable diaper with the plastic outer covering. The humidity in there is 100 percent. This makes a magnificent culture medium for the growth of yeast, which is normally found in a baby's diaper area. This yeast then grows and invades the tender skin of your baby's bottom, making a red, itchy, scaly, sometimes weeping and bleeding irritation of the skin.

The problem has been greatly compounded over the last few years with the advent of disposable diapers with elastic around the leg band areas so that no moisture can escape.

Another problem with the diaper area is the use of thick ointments on a baby as a more or less continuous form of "protection" of the tender groin areas. Babies have been brought into my office so thickly coated with ointment and baby powder that it has taken half an hour to scrub all the goo from the skin so that I could see the rash!

If you want to cleanse your baby's bottom, do it with a nice mild soap like Dove, and use a mild anti-yeast, drying powder like Caldesene. Never use ointments unless your doctor prescribes them.

So the "bottom" line on diaper dermatitis is this: Use paper disposable diapers judiciously (or not at all) if your baby has any tendency toward diaper rash. Keep it simple. Clean the child with a mild soap and maybe you won't have your neighbors and parents asking if your child is really a little lobster.

TOPICALS FOR INFANTS

Early in dermatology training, we are told to listen carefully to pediatricians when they make comments about the skin. Why? Because pediatricians get to see so much skin and so many skin problems that they become excellent dermatologists over the years. Some advocate the routine use of baby oil and/or baby powder on the skin of infants. But unless your child has a problem, there is no real need to put baby oil on his or her skin. If your child has a dry, scaly skin rash, it is certainly harmless to try baby oil as a type of moisturizer for a while, and I think most of us in dermatology, and certainly most mothers and pediatricians, would agree that baby powder is fairly harmless and a very pleasant substance to use. I can remember times when I was a child getting out of a bathtub, drying well, and then being doused thoroughly with baby powder. It always felt very good and never caused any problem. Use it if you like. But remember to put the powder in your hand and smoothe it on the baby gently, so the child doesn't breathe in the powder.

If you ever have the opportunity to look at baby powder under a microscope you will see that the talc in the powder looks like tiny jagged pieces of glass under magnification. It's really hard to imagine how such a substance could be put on soft baby skin without being irritating. But in fact, the jagged edges of the talc flakes must be compensated for by the incredible smoothness and flatness of the tiny plates of powder. The theory is that even though the edges are somewhat jagged, the flakes actually do glide over one another very smoothly.

I don't think much of cornstarch powders. Cornstarch has been known to support yeast growth, which, as you already know, is a chronic source of diaper rash and irritation. Therefore, if you want a good powder, use Caldesene. It's available in a pink can in the baby section of drugstores. This agent has talc, but it also has an anti-yeast substance that can help prevent diaper rash in your child.

Premoistened paper wipes are safe to use at diaper changes provided the infant shows no allergic reaction to them. (However, I've never known anyone to encounter such problems.)

Beards and Shaving

Sometimes male teens complain that their beards are not filling out the way they'd like them to. But beard growth is determined by individual sets of genes. They tell it when to start and where to grow. And there's not much a person can do about making it grow where it doesn't want to. But taking a close look at uncles on both sides of the family and at Dad will give some idea of what one's permanent beard pattern will be.

Many men (and women, for that matter) believe that shaving stimulates hair growth. This is completely false! If it were true, bald men would be shaving their heads a couple of times daily to see if they could get hair to grow!

Birthmarks

A birthmark is a spot on the skin that is present on the person's day of birth. There are many types of birthmarks, and they are often lifelong problems.

Why is it that some of us are born with faultless, unsmudged skin, and others are born with birthmarks? We just don't know. We do know that some types of moles are heritable, but we have very little information on the origins of other types.

Chance? Genetics? Some developmental accident? Drugs? Toxins? Maybe all or none. A study in *Clinical Pediatrics* (August 1978) showed that 21 percent of children with hemangiomas (the red type) had a definite family history of them. That's much higher than the population in general and does indeed indicate that heredity plays some part in their development.

Some birthmarks represent serious problems, occasionally even life-threatening ones; others are lifelong stains. that can affect every facet of one's life. Let's consider the various types separately.

CAFÉ AU LAIT SPOTS

Some babies are born with brown flat spots on their skin. Some of these spots do not appear until the child is several months old. Some of these are *café au lait* spots (French for "coffee with milk"; these spots actually do have this shading). Such children should be examined by a dermatologist. The child may have other skin conditions and even internal problems related to the skin spot that should be discussed with your dermatologist.

One patient's mother asked if it was the silver nitrate put in the child's eyes at birth that caused this discoloration. It was not. Silver nitrate discoloration is superficial, does not usually occur with the eyedrops, and occurs within hours of the exposure, not months.

I can't adequately explain why marks sometimes appear at one month of age or later. Many of the pigmented spots do, however, gradually darken during infancy and childhood.

Note that if your child does have a *café au lait* spot, it can be masked much more easily than some of the darker spots we will talk about in succeeding sections.

HAIRY BIRTHMARKS

Brown, raised, hairy moles represent a completely different type of birthmark. For years it was thought that these moles were benign and could be left alone because they never turned into skin cancers. The exception to this was the large "bathing trunk nevus," which covered widespread areas on the back in the bathing suit area. These often developed into a very serious life-threatening form of skin cancer called malignant melanoma. One study, in the 1977 *Scandinavian Journal of Plastic and Reconstructive Surgery*, indicates that 5 percent of them turn into fatal melanomas. I will have more to say about malignant melanoma in a later chapter.

In the wake of years of observation by skin cancer experts, dermatologists have come to the conclusion that these moles, thought so long to be no problem to the children who have them, should often be removed. It is estimated that some 7 to 17 percent of them, if they are dark brown and were present on the day of the child's birth, will turn into malignant melanoma at some time during the child's life. Usually this malignant degeneration occurs before the late teens, though it can occur at any time.

So dermatologists who study these congenital melanocytic nevi, as they are called, often suggest early removal as the best possible course. In the 1977 Scandinavian study, every child whose mole turned to melanoma died. Naturally, it is a huge task for a surgeon to remove very large lesions from the back and the buttocks. But it should and can be done with the advice and help of a plastic surgeon.

If the moles are small, they can easily be taken off and closed primarily, that is, with a simple line of stitches, right in the doctor's office. However, the larger lesions sometimes require removal in strips and often may require skin grafts to cover the defect. Plastic surgeons usually do the larger mole removals, but some dermatologists (who are also dermatologic surgeons) can do this procedure.

PORT-WINE STAINS

The story of red birthmarks is one of the most heart-rending chapters in dermatologic history. The conventional term for this type of spot is port-wine stain (PWS), or nevus flammeus. The term originated in the 1800s when, in England, physicians noticed that spills of port wine on tablecloths looked like the color of the nevus flammeus.

Today, while we still don't know the cause of PWS spots, we do know some things that should be done for them, and some things that should not be done.

Port-wine stains are collections of dilated, or widely opened superficial blood veins, or capillaries, which often appear at birth or a few months thereafter. They are a lot darker and redder than the "salmon patch," which is a lighter birthmark usually over the back, upper neck, and glabellar area of the forehead (the small triangle over the nasal bridge area). Port-wine stains usually start out as slightly pink spots that get slowly redder through childhood and darken into a deep wine red in adolescence and early adulthood. They actually turn frankly purple and bumpy in middle and old age. They can sometimes cover the entire length of the leg or occasionally half the body.

Sometimes these spots can cause massive swelling of the tissues in the areas occupied by the lesions. This can result in enlargement of the bones and body structures below these spots.

Folk tales about the origins of birthmarks are amazing. One patient told me that her mother accounted for this by telling her that, while her mother was pregnant, a neighbor's house caught fire. She says her mother put her hand to the right side of her face in fear and terror, and that's what caused her mark. But scientifically, there's no way at all that the fire tragedy had anything to do with that spot.

There have been hundreds of different treatments tried for PWS throughout the history of medicine. For years small ones were cut off and the defect was sewn shut, producing a scar of variable size and length. This worked fairly well for small spots if the patient could tolerate the scar that results, but for large spots, and for those spots that involve vital structures such as the eyelid, there is no way to do this surgery without leaving a mark that looks much worse than the PWS. Cryosurgery (freezing) has been tried with very little success, and so has tattooing the lesions with flesh-colored ink. This latter can occasionally dull the tone of the redness, but the look is usually unsatisfactory.

Over the last fifteen years, however, a "new light" has appeared on the horizon for those with PWS. That light is the laser. This is truly one of the great success stories in medicine, since the technique works best in those lesions that are the worst: purple, dark, nodular marks on the face.

Pioneered by dermatologist Dr. Leon Goldman of the University of Cincinnati and followed up by the highly skilled Laser Treatment Unit of Beth-Israel Hospital in Boston, Massachusetts, laser therapy means great relief from a stigma that can literally destroy one's life.

This therapy is most effective for those who are over seventeen years old and who have deep-red to purple and even nodular lesions. Regrettably, it does not work as well in the very young and/or in those with pink or light-red lesions. This is unfortunate for the young because the lightening of these spots could result in a much more relaxed and successful childhood.

Laser treatment for PWS, however, is difficult and somewhat painful. Usually more than one treatment is required, and there is no guarantee that the mark will be completely erased. Frankly, complete removal is often not possible. The laser surgeon's aim is to decrease the defect as much as possible. The laser treatments can involve scarring. However, this is very infrequent and usually occurs in specific areas of the head and neck.

The treatment works even on eyelids, a fact that makes it the most effective and advanced form of spot removal for this location.

If you have a port-wine stain that is annoying or causing significant problems for you, discuss it with your dermatologist and ask for a referral to a center for laser treatment. Many dermatologists in private practice are now highly skilled in the use of the laser. Many different types of laser exist for treating various colors of spots, so careful consultation is required to establish whether or not laser therapy could be effective in each child's case.

PWS patients should keep in mind, however, that their skin markings may be with them throughout life. They should also keep in mind that their friends will accept them because they are their friends. Remember, too, that even if the marks cannot be removed, there are ways to disguise them.

THE COVERMARK AND DERMABLEND SYSTEMS

Lydia O'Leary designed the Covermark makeup system in the late 1930s to be used over port-wine stains. It's so dramatically effective in PWS lesions that dermatologists themselves sometimes find it nearly undetectable. I first saw the Covermark system demonstrated at an American Academy of Dermatology meeting several years ago. A very pleasant lady was showing all the techniques used for covering port-wine stains and other lesions. She showed a picture of a young woman who somehow looked quite familiar to me but had an incredible dark-purple port-wine stain covering half her face. In the next picture, this same lady's face was completely "free" of this gigantic deforming lesion. It was then that I realized where I had seen the lady in this picture. It was a picture of the lady showing the very pictures we were looking at! Standing in front of me was the same lady some ten years older than she was in the picture but wearing her Covermark cosmetics, so that I had not even suspected she had the PWS problem.

She went on to demonstrate the various techniques for effectively covering all types of skin blemishes, including unsightly enlarged veins on the legs. Since that time I have prescribed Covermark cosmetics for blemishes of every shape, size, and description. The system has worked well for nearly all these patients.

Covermark Cosmetics
330 Washington Avenue
Carlstadt, NJ 07072
1-800-424-1120

You may contact them for brochures regarding the availability of Covermark cosmetics and their other products in your area.

The other system for covering severe marks on the skin is called Dermablend. This cosmetic system is as widely available as is

Covermark, and often larger department stores have experts on staff who have been trained in the application of these cover-up cosmetics, so you should call around to your favorite store to find out. Often, the dermatologists in any one area may know which stores sell these two brands. They may be tough to find, but they are certainly worth the trouble. You can also write to the following address:

Dermablend Corrective Makeup
852 South Layfette Avenue
Chicago, IL 60620

STRAWBERRY MARKS

Strawberry birthmarks are small, bright-red collections of abnormally growing blood vessels that usually increase in size slightly during the first year or so of life. After this time they will usually become stable or start to regress.

To remember best the natural course of a strawberry birthmark, you should remember the numbers 5, 7, and 9. The 5 stands for the fact that 50 percent of these lesions are gone completely by the age of 5, 70 percent are usually gone by the age of 7, and 90 percent are gone by the age of 9. While this does not hold as a hard and fast rule by any means, it is generally true that most of the lesions resolve spontaneously.

If your child is bothered by the presence of a red mark, as could be expected, you should know several things about treatment. First, try not to treat it! The naturally resolved strawberry mark is nearly invisible. However, almost anything done to these marks can leave a scar or permanent defect that later can look much worse than if it had been left alone. This is especially true for conventional surgical removal in which the marks look worse nearly every time. However, sometimes an early resolution can be initiated by a very light spray with liquid nitrogen, a freezing technique called cryosurgery.

In some children these strawberry lesions begin to grow rapidly after birth and can obstruct a vital organ such as the air passage in the throat, or they can interfere with sight if they are near an eye. In these cases most dermatologists would choose to treat the child with large doses of cortisone to slow and reverse the growth of the spot. This method is not to be taken lightly, however, since cortisone has long-term side effects in some patients. It is advisable, therefore, to use this only with infants who have severe lesions.

There are several angiomatous, or blood-vessel-type lesions that could occur in infants. If they are getting larger it would be wise to use the cortisone treatment now because they will sometimes continue to get larger throughout infancy. But don't have them removed surgically, as I have said before, until they are evaluated by a dermatologist.

DON'T BE CAUGHT WITH A RED FACE

Do you have a chronically red nose and cannot, for some reason, have laser therapy? Try green "color correction foundation." That's right, I said green! The reason behind this is simple: When the red on your nose and the makeup's green color combine, a flesh tone is produced. The color corrector is available at most cosmetic counters, and there are several other manufacturers who produce a green-tinted foundation.

There are other causes of redness on the face from the expansion of small facial blood vessels. Most of us in dermatology feel the sun causes redness by enlarging otherwise tiny vessels. We also know that the use of certain topical compounds for treatment of some skin problems of the face can make them appear. These topicals, called fluorinated steroids, are forms of cortisone with an attached fluoride molecule. The fluoride makes the creams about ten times more potent, but the subsequent higher potency can both induce thinning in the skin and cause tiny blood vessels to grow quite large. Therefore, I'm constantly on the lookout for patients using treatment creams that are fluorinated. Except in the most dire circumstances, they're rarely needed on the soft skin of the face, neck, groin, or other soft-skin areas.

Black Skin

SOME GOOD NEWS AND SOME BAD NEWS

Black skin is a magnificent organ that contains its own sun protection, the pigment melanin. This brownish-black pigment is produced in a host of tiny pigment cells called melanocytes lying in an almost unbroken layer along the bottom cell layer of the epidermis. In some areas there are virtually thousands per square centimeter. The pigment they produce is an incredible sunshield! It's so effective, in fact, that sun-induced skin cancer is extraordinarily rare among blacks, and wrinkling is greatly retarded too.

Amazingly, there are about the same number of pigment-producing melanocytes in black and in white skin. In blacks, however, the melanocytes crank out more melanin and melanin of different types than that secreted by Caucasians.

Melanocytes are very responsive cells. Sunlight and all kinds of other injuries can make them turn on like little factories to crank out mountains of pigment when it's needed (and, as we shall see, sometimes when it's not!).

So the good news is that black skin is resistant to skin cancer. It's also slightly less likely to contract contact allergy. What about Asian-type skin? In Asians, the actual molecular type of melanin and the distribution of the pigment are different. Dr. Ken Hashimoto, Chairman of Dermatology at Wayne State University, says that major surveys have been done in the Japanese population. "Asians have very rare basal cell carcinomas and rare premalignant actinic keratoses (sunspots). In this sense, oriental skin is more resistant to skin cancer than is Caucasian skin, but somewhat less resistant to skin cancer than black skin."

Renowned dermatologist Ernst Epstein goes even further in stating that he cannot remember (in his extensive experience) ever seeing a melanoma in an Asian patient. He is quick to caution that he is sure they occur, but in his practice, he's not seen them.

Black skin, however, has some special problems. Among those problems more prevalent in blacks is a serious one called razor dermatitis.

BEARD BUMPS (RAZOR DERMATITIS)

Many blacks have problems with shaving in the neck area, including sensitivity to shaving preparations that irritate the skin. Often this problem is like an acne eruption in the bearded areas. This is a very annoying condition called pseudofolliculitis barbae, or PFB. PFB (razor dermatitis or razor bumps) is an inflammation or irritation produced where curly beard hairs repenetrate the facial and neck skin, causing inflammation or soreness. Note that the irritation is not where the hairs come out of the skin (the hair follicle), but at the site of repenetration. That's why it's called pseudo-, or false, folliculitis. While this occurs very commonly in blacks, some curly-haired whites also have the problem.

Shaving is the definitive cause of PFB, so that stopping shaving brings about a very rapid improvement. The worst thing that patients can do is to continue shaving.

We have known for a long time that the definitive cure for PFB is growing a beard. While the beard is coming out we encourage the men to flip out these small, repenetrating hairs (called "bucket handles") from the skin where they are growing back in. This can be done with a toothpick and allows the beard to grow without curling hairs up inside the skin. If circumstances prohibit the growing of a beard, which is often the case for people in business and in the military, we ask patients to wash the facial area with a Buf-Puf and a mild soap. Then the skin is well dried and various medications can be applied. These include topical antibiotics and anti-acne preparations such as vitamin A acid (Retin-A) and benzoyl peroxide. A word should also be said about the type of razor used. The worst of all possible razors is the double-track razor. With this twin-bladed razor, the first blade cuts off the hair and the second blade often slices off a small bump of skin below the hair. This causes secondary infection and scarring and facilitates repenetration of the hair back into the skin. An electric razor is still the least traumatic for the skin. If a person decides he cannot tolerate a beard and he uses an electric razor, a light oil preshave, such as Williams' 'Lectric Shave, may be used so that the surface of the razor will glide more easily.

KELOIDS—SCARS GONE WILD

Thickened, tender scars are called keloids. Keloids are very common in blacks, less common in olive-skinned people, and rare in Caucasians. Minor keloids are called hypertrophic (overgrown) scars, but keloids themselves go further than just simple enlargement. They grow out of and away from their natural boundaries and extend to normal skin.

In blacks, they start out as a reddish scar that swells up above the surrounding skin and gets progressively harder. As time passes, they acquire a brownish pigmentation and then usually darken intensely to a skin tone several shades deeper than the usual skin color for the area.

Although surgical wounds are the most common sites where keloids develop, they do occur in many other types of injury such as acne lesions, cuts, scrapes, and burns.

If you are facing sugery, you should mention to your doctor whether you or your family are prone to forming these scars. This is helpful to know before surgery, so that some precautions can be taken. For instance, many doctors will anesthetize the surgical site with a numbing medicine mixed with cortisone so that it's less likely to heal with a big scar.

Pierced ears account for the majority of keloids in my practice, and they're one of the biggest headaches to get rid of, too. Of course, pierced ears are the rage in our society, so it's unlikely that I could convince people not to have the piercing procedure done, but black women deserve a special note of caution. Unfortunately, I've seen ear keloids as big as a walnut on black patients. This ear-piercing operation can cause keloids to form regardless of who does the piercing. And once the keloid forms, it's very difficult, if not impossible, to get rid of it.

Most ear piercing is done in a department store by nonmedical personnel. That means that you may have problems with infection and nickel allergy, as well as with scarring. Were this not so, do you think they'd make you sign that long form prior to your piercing operation? I don't stand alone when I say that surgery should be done only by surgeons. That means that lay persons, no matter what training they have, are unlikely to be able to adequately advise you on the possible complications of the procedure.

Ordinarily, with a lump or bump somewhere, you'd just expect the surgeon to excise the lesion. In keloids, however, that often results in the regrowth of the lesion to an even bigger size. Treatment often involves the use of cortisone injections and also radiation therapy to control subsequent scarring. Sometimes, even with these treatments, the keloids still come back larger than they were originally. You can see that keloids are not an easy problem. Cortisone injections often clear up the itching in keloids in just a few days. Topical cortisone creams also help itching, but you should be careful to apply the medicine only to the keloid to prevent the medicine from thinning the skin around it.

Gallbladder scars also often turn out badly because there is so much tension on that area of the abdominal skin that they stretch and spread very easily. Revision by a plastic surgeon engenders the same risks as revision of the scars on the earlobes caused by piercing. However, you should consult your local plastic surgeon. He or she will tell you, after an examination and after taking your history, whether or not surgery would result in a successful revision of the scar.

CORNROW HAIR LOSS

Some black children wear tight braids in their hair, known as "cornrowing." Sometimes, the hair thins in between the rows. We see all too much of this problem, called traction alopecia. It's a real hazard for blacks who desire to have the new plaited hairstyles, especially the very fine braids, because these braids exert fantastic traction, or pulling stresses, on the scalp hairs.

With this chronic pulling of the hairs, scarring is induced deep down in the follicle where the hair is made. This results in the gradual obliteration of the active hair-growing apparatus and, with it, permanent hair loss. This is the same kind of process that results in loss of hair in nurses who pin on their caps so tightly that they begin to lose hair over the years.

Traction alopecia can be a true disaster if it's not recognized and stopped quickly. Braiding of the hair does not have to stop altogether, but at least the tension on the base of the hairs where they are attached to the scalp should be lessened. Start braiding very loosely so that almost no tension is put on the scalp skin. Ask your daughter to tell you when and if it begins to feel tight. Often the child can tell the tightness a lot better than the mother can. Cornrowing is okay, but do it right and avoid possible permanent hair loss.

DARKER SPOTS

Through the pigment in black skin is protective, it can be a problem when deposited in excess, causing darker brown spots on the skin. Remember the tiny color cells, or melanocytes? These diminutive pigment factories are most efficient producers of brown pigment, and usually they do it in a very regular, controlled fashion. This gives the skin an even brownish to black coloration. However, any physical trauma can greatly stimulate the output of melanin, causing the skin to darken drastically in just a matter of days.

There are two components to this pigment darkening—an epidermal, or surface darkening and a dermal, or deeper darkening. The epidermal type of pigment will usually resolve with time. The dermal deposits, however, are another story. They are not likely to lighten to normal skin tone very quickly, if at all. Sometimes it takes years for this type of stain to lighten significantly. In rare cases, the spots are permanent, just like tattoos.

Hypermelanosis, as the spots of extra dark pigment are called, is best treated by "tincture of time" therapy. That is, most dermatologists would choose to wait for the spots to improve naturally before resorting to a pigment lightener. Among the available lighteners is Melanex, which also treats melasma, the mask of pregnancy. It's a prescription drug available only through your doctor. The addition of Retin-A powder to Melanex can be beneficial in speeding the pigment resolution.

Of critical importance is halting or ameliorating whatever caused the darkening in the first place. I'll give you an example. Sylvia, a black patient with acne, had discovered that a loofah sponge made her facial skin feel soft and smooth. She liked the feel of it so much that she started using her loofah three or four times a day. She forgot how harsh these scrubbers are and soon noticed some pigment darkening on her face that she tried even harder to scrub away. Sylvia realized too late that the dark spots, now huge brown-black triangles on her face, were actually caused by the scrubbing process.

I stopped Sylvia's use of the loofah and put her on antibiotics for her acne. She began to clear quite rapidly, but the total time to achieve normal skin color was over ten months. So if you have black skin, be careful with it. It'll pigment at the slightest provocation.

Bruising

Almost everyone gets some blue-black bruising on the backs of their hands and arms if they live long enough. These spots, previously called senile purpura (a horrible term), are now referred to as ecchymoses (eck-ee-MO-sees), or superficial bruises. There are several reasons why we tend to get these when we grow older. First and foremost, the skin thins as aging occurs, causing the strong support network of collagen in the skin to weaken. This weakening allows the tiny blood vessels in the upper skin layers to break at the slightest tap. Also, sunlight seems to play a part in the weakening of these vessels. They seem to be much more common in sun-exposed people than in others.

There is no real way to prevent ecchymoses from happening. The only way I've been able to help patients with them is to advise the persons to be extraordinarily careful about trauma on their arms. And if they do see an ecchymosis developing after a minor injury, keep firm pressure on the exact spot where the injury took place for about five to seven minutes. This allows the blood to clot in the wall of the injured blood vessel, stopping further leakage. At least the pressure technique can prevent the ecchymoses from getting too large.

One more important fact about ecchymoses—the chronic, repeated deposition of blood under the skin will often leave a brownish discoloration in the skin substance itself. That's why it's important to try to prevent these lesions. Use my "firm pressure" method and you'll see results.

The fact that you get ecchymoses in your seventies does not necessarily mean that you have a blood disease. However, any serious bleeding tendency, especially if not localized to the arms, should be evaluated by your doctor. He or she may want to do clotting tests and other tests on your blood and look for internal diseases.

Experts also caution that people with the problem should not take any aspirin unless directed to do so for some other medical problem. Aspirin causes easy bruising by stopping the aggregation of the body's platelets, an essential clotting factor.

Sometimes from time to time some elderly people have actual tears in the skin, leaving scars behind to heal with whitish discolorations. A lot of older people get these, quite innocently, when they apply tape to their arms. The simple removal of the tape can cause a serious rip in the delicate skin of the arms. Never apply adhesive tape to the arms of the elderly, if it can be avoided. All bandages needed in the area of the thin skin of the arms should be wrapped gently with gauze bandages.

Petechiae are tiny blood hemorrhages in the very uppermost layer of the skin. There is a variety of causes of these lesions, from just being normal to having leukemia or lymphoma. Your doctor will want to thoroughly rule out serious medical diseases, and he or she may choose to send off a skin biopsy to see, on a microscopic level, what's actually going on in the skin. Sometimes various irritations of the blood vessels, called vasculitis, can be found in this manner. Then the exact causes of the vasculitis must be sought with detailed testing. It's not only the elderly who get petechiae, so anyone with red spots should get them looked at.

Cellulite

GREAT INTERNATIONAL HOAX

"Cellulite" is the greatest dermatologic hoax ever perpetrated on the beauty-conscious American public. The very term "cellulite" even sounds like one's cells are contaminated with some modern pollutant. Cellulite is just a descriptive term for the way fat piles up in the supporting network of the skin. The more fat, the more dimples! The less fat, the less dimples. It's really as simple as that, but every time I tell audiences about the truth of the horrible and dreaded cellulite, I receive calls and letters by the hundreds, telling me what an iconoclast and beauty nihilist I am. Sorry, but truth's truth. Okay, then, what would one do to stop getting it? Stop eating.

FAT SUCTION—NOT NECESSARILY THE "EASY" WAY

Can you lose cellulite by having the fat suction operation? On a television talk show I once said the best cure for cellulite was weight loss. Then I got a letter from a fairly thin woman with the problem who had, in about two months, gained ten pounds. Then the cellulite started to show up on her upper thighs. What to do to get rid of this ugly stuff, besides losing weight? How about the new "suction" operation for this?

In this operation, fat cells are sucked out through a tube inserted in the skin through a small inconspicuous incision. While the technique definitely has merit, I'd hasten to add that some very severe complications can result. These include infection below the skin, hemorrhage, and disruption of the nerves, arteries, and veins that supply the involved skin.

Ask your plastic surgeon specifically about his or her special competence in the suction operation: total number of cases, results, complications, photos of his or her actual real patients, and, most important, a list of patients your surgeon has operated on so you can talk to them personally and actually see the results.

Corns

and Footwear

AH, THERE'S THE RUB!

One of the most annoying conditions we see in the office is that of "soft corns." These are painfully thickened skin between the fourth and fifth toes, almost always in women. A wonderful podiatrist who had treated my mother's soft corns used to say, "The poor feet! Whenever you realize you have feet, there's almost always something wrong with them!" And he was right. Tight footwear is the main reason for the formation of soft corns. It seems that in the search for fashion we've created several new diseases, not the least of which are these nasty little nuisances called "soft corns."

Whenever two toes are pushed together, as they are most effectively with tight footwear, the skin begins to thicken to protect and cushion the bones below. But the poor skin, just doing its faithful job of protecting our innards, doesn't realize that the thickening will eventually hurt and greatly irritate the skin itself. Correction of the problem depends on relieving the pressure of the narrow footwear while treating the corns. Treating them is much easier said than done, however. Some people can get relief by just putting cotton pads, or even "doughnut"-type adhesive bandages around the corns to better distribute the pressure over a larger area. Often, however, it's necessary to use a mild salicylic acid plaster (available at foot-care counters) to soften and gently coax the thick part of the corn off the tender skin below. Follow the directions on the package very carefully, especially the advice concerning diabetic foot care, because no diabetic should undergo any foot treatment without his or her doctor's advice.

Cosmetics

"SKIN WRITING"—BLACK DERMATOGRAPHISM

I have many women patients who tell me about an unusual problem. They buy good jewelry, but constantly have black discolorations of the skin under the metal frames of their glasses where they touch their cheeks and under their rings, which are made of silver and gold. Often they think they create chemicals in their skins that cause this problem specifically. To me, this is one of the most fascinating stories in all of dermatology. First, it doesn't happen just to an occasional woman, but to thousands of women. Second, no skin chemical is responsible for this discoloration. Third, their silver and gold rings probably are the fine metals they think they are. The real problem is, remarkably, their face powder.

Let me explain. Jewelry metals are usually fairly soft. But face powders contain extremely hard, tiny, sharp flakes of metals such as titanium, which are much harder than the metals in your jewelry. The friction of glass rims upon the powder on the cheeks and of the rings on the fingers of the hands that applied the powder actually causes infinitesimal particles of gold or silver to be abraded from both glasses and rings. Why doesn't the abraded metal look gold or silver in color, then? Because the particles are so tiny that they won't accurately reflect light much at all. They just scatter it. Therefore, taken together, they look black. And for that reason, the problem has been named black dermatographism, which means "black-colored skin writing."

So how does a woman get around this unsightly problem? Simple! Try not to get any powder on the cheek areas that contact the rims of your glasses. And don't fail to wash your hands thoroughly after each use of your face powder. The problem will leave you instantly.

Cysts

BREAST SKIN CYSTS

Occasionally a woman will develop a few plugged oil glands around the areolae, or brown areas of the nipples, usually in response to nursing an infant. These are quite normal if they're not excessively large and sometimes will go away without treatment. If they get large, sore, inflamed, or infected, they should be examined by a physician. Antibiotics, surgery, or a combination may be needed to resolve them. Diet has nothing to do with the development of these tiny cysts.

Dandruff

NOTHING STOPS DANDRUFF
LIKE A DARK-BLUE SUIT!

"Just look at this," said Candace as she moved her long brown hair off her dandruff-speckled sweater, "have you ever seen it this bad before? I keep hoping it'll snow every day, so people won't know about my problem."

When I looked at all the scales on her shoulders, I was reminded of my mentor, Dr. Glenn Marsh, who used to say, "Nothing stops dandruff like a dark-blue suit!" In fact, Candace had not been able to wear blue for years, because of her dandruff.

What would you say if I told you everybody's got to have dandruff? Yep! That's right! Everybody. If we didn't, our scalps would be ten feet thick! You see, the skin remakes itself from top to bottom every twenty-eight days, so all that dead stuff's got to go somewhere. That's what the flakes are. The actual process is called seborrhea, or running of oil.

We think that scalp oil irritates the surface of the skin after it's secreted. As a parallel, consider stomach acid. If stomach acid remains in the stomach, no harm done. But if the acid regurgitates into the esophagus, or food tube, we feel the burning irritation as "heartburn." The situation is similar with dandruff and the worse form, seborrheic (seb-oh-REE-ick) dermatitis. The sebaceous oil is nonirritating while it's inside the oil gland, but does in fact irritate when it lies upon the scalp.

I'm constantly amazed, in my day-to-day practice of dermatology, how many people feel that washing the hair is somehow harmful. It's not. In fact, most people don't wash their hair enough to keep the oil removed efficiently. Amazingly, I've had numbers of patients who wash their hair only every two weeks or less, and a few who, because of especially difficult hair styles, wash only once monthly! Imagine the tremendous amount of oil that is held onto or near the scalp. This much scalp oil can be very irritating.

69

Seborrheic dermatitis is accompanied by scalp irritation and redness with severe scaling. It takes special medications, including more potent tar shampoos and often topical cortisone, to get this under control. The odor is caused by bacteria that build up in the excess scalp oil characteristic of this condition. It's most effectively relieved by frequent washing, usually once daily.

Seborrheic dermatitis often starts in the late teens and early twenties. It's much more common in men than in women. Often it spreads from the scalp to the sides of the nose, eyebrows, and even the breast-line area.

If scales "stick more to the scalp," the condition might be psoriasis. Be sure to read about this elsewhere in this book to find out all about it.

TREATMENTS FOR SEBORRHEIC DERMATITIS

Treatment of this scaly, itchy scalp condition has changed somewhat in recent years. It is now realized that a superficial yeast growth on the scalp may be the activating factor, along with a person's natural oiliness, of seborrheic dermatitis. This discovery prompted the use of anti-yeast preparations, first on the scaly red areas of the face and then in the development of an anti-yeast shampoo called Nizoral. At this time, in my office, almost every patient with recognizable seborrhea or seborrheic dermatitis gets a prescription for Nizoral cream and/or shampoo. The cream is used once or twice daily, and the shampoo should be used twice weekly for five to seven minutes in order to kill off these needless and itch-causing yeast organisms.

I encourage the use of mild- and moderate-strength tar shampoos on the days when Nizoral shampoo is not being used. More about these later.

A word about "pH balance" of shampoos; pH is an indicator of acidity. A low pH shampoo is more acid and theoretically is better for your hair. I would search for a fairly low pH shampoo, such as Ionil T Plus, if I had seborrheic dermatitis, because not only does it have a nice low pH, but the tar and salicylic acid in it are extremely effective scale removers in seborrhea and seborrheic dermatitis. If you don't have a particular scalp condition, Phacid is the all-time best and mildest shampoo.

Flaky ears with a lot of itching is a regular characteristic of seborrheic dermatitis. But it can also happen in psoriasis and other diseases, so be sure to check with your dermatologist to make sure.

One of the main conditions we worry about in the ears, when they've been treated with multiple medicines, is allergic contact dermatitis. That is, it's possible to be allergic to one or more of the ingredients of the medicines used for ear canal problems.

Be sure to read the discussion of the treatment of ear canals in the psoriasis section, "Beating Psoriasis—How to Live Without Leaving a Trail of Scales." The technique that employs Halog or Lidex solution on a Q-tip is the most effective I've ever found for handling ear canal rashes.

Seborrheic dermatitis is not a contagious disease. Beauty shop patrons do not have to be fearful of "catching" the disease. Seborrheic dermatitis is no more contagious than freckles or a big nose.

Now that you realize that all scalps have dandruff, you'll be better equipped to seek help if the condition progresses. With the shampoos and medicines available today, no one needs to put up with "snowy shoulders." If your scaling and itching problem is severe, relief is as close as your dermatologist's office.

Dry Skin

WINTER ITCH

It was another freezing January day in Lexington. Winter was taking its usual heavy toll on skin. My first patient of the day was bent over, scratching and digging at her legs.

"Dr. Bark, you've got to help me," said the frustrated patient. "My family has threatened to move me into the basement if I don't quit scratching my legs!" She pulled up a pant leg to reveal a shin loaded with tiny bleeding cracks I recognized immediately as winter dry skin.

"How many times per day do you bathe?" I asked, anticipating her answer.

"Well, usually two, but the water makes my legs feel so good! It's later that they seem to itch so much."

"Aha! You've hit squarely on the problem. But you're really making the problem worse. Now let's see if a few modifications in your routine can improve your condition."

Winter after winter dermatologists hear such complaints of dry-skin problems. And while dryness can strike any age group, it's much more common as one ages. It's really true that our oil gland output drops sharply after our teens. This decrease in oiliness plus winter dry air can lead straight to a case of severe dry skin. But it's possible to live with smooth, supple skin even if you're not a teenager and even in winter. This section will teach you the secrets that dermatologists use to correct almost any dry-skin problem.

THE GENESIS OF DRY SKIN

The condition of dryness of the skin is called xerosis. This is a term derived from a Greek word meaning "dryness." It should not be confused in name with psoriasis, the scaly red genetic skin disease, or cirrhosis, a disease of inflammation and hardening of the liver. Xerosis is a very common, noninfectious disease that occurs with greater frequency during the fall and winter months because of the low humidity. In fact, many people call xerosis "winter itch" because during periods of low humidity, the skin dries out horribly. The condition is usually found in areas of the body where oil glands are not very numerous, such as the arms, legs, and trunk areas.

When the skin dries out, the dead top layer of the skin stiffens and cracks. This cracking causes fissures in the skin, which then become irritated, inflamed, and very itchy. This problem is by no means confined to one age group or sex. It is found in young children, as well as in middle-aged and elderly adults. Even teenagers can get it on nonoily parts of their skin.

There are many contributing factors to xerosis besides the season of the year. The second most common cause is the use of harsh antibacterial soaps. Some patients find that they contribute to dry skin. The newer liquid soaps in dispenser bottles are also extremely drying. In fact, many of these soaps contain substances that, during the summer months, can even react with sunlight striking the skin, causing an itchy eruption on the skin, which is very serious. We'll talk about the right soap to use in a minute.

The next most common cause of xerosis is excess bathing. Television and commercial advertisements have made us all too conscious of the "need" for frequent skin cleansing. Repeated washing removes the skin's natural oil layer. This allows evaporation of the skin's water, which, in turn, leaves the very substance of the skin dry. In other words, water and bathing are extremely drying to the skin. As a matter of fact, xerosis is only a product of recent years, because people never used to take as many baths as they do now, and if they only took one bath a week (whether they needed it or not), they had a chance to reaccumulate their natural body oils in between baths. Then they just didn't have dry skin.

What can you do about your extremely dry skin? Decrease your baths to a maximum of one every other day, if possible. If you find it necessary to bathe in between your baths, just spot-baths. Usually, Dove (found in two studies to be the mildest soap), used in small amounts, is perfectly adequate for cleansing. If you cannot use it for any reason, then use Lowila, Basis, or Neutrogena soap.

The whole principle of bathing and soap use can be summed up by using the "three gits": "Git in, git clean, and git out!"

After bathing, it's absolutely crucial that you replace the oil you've washed off your skin. I prefer that you use a bath oil after each bath or shower, but do not follow the directions on the bottle. The instructions tell you to put the oil into the water. Never put bath oil in your bath water. This is wasteful because the bath oil, for the most part, goes down the drain instead of onto your skin.

The oil also makes the tub extremely slippery. So, to avoid both problems (losing most of your bath oil and slipping on it), you should apply the bath oil to your wet skin while standing outside the tub. You may then pat dry gently, but do not rub off the oil you've just applied.

Dry-skin lotions have come a long way in 3,000 years, since the Egyptian women first used scented oils to coat their skin after bathing. That was really the first generation of moisturizers.

Second-generation moisturizers came along in the 1940s with the advent of oil-in-water emulsions. These moisturizers really just contained a lot of water and some oil to layer over the skin and seal in the water. This worked pretty well, but the skin still lost fantastic amounts of water through insensible loss, that is, the daily water evaporation of which none of us is aware.

In the 1970s, urea was added to the later second-generation moisturizers. Urea is a hygroscopic material, meaning it actually draws water into the skin and holds it there. The only trouble with urea was its tendency to sting when applied to tender areas of the skin.

That left the door open for the third generation of moisturizers, those with alpha hydroxy acids. These acids, namely glycolic, lactic, and a few others, are tremendous moisteners of the skin. At the same time they remove some of the rough dead skin cells from the dry surface of the skin so that we don't look so scaly in the winter time. Some very excellent lotions are Lacticare, LacHydrin-5, and Moisturel Lotion as well as Aveeno Lotion and Eucerin Lotion, the last two being heavier than the others, for more difficult cases.

In the winter, you have several options open to you for your lips. Most women who wear lipstick do just fine with only that, if they wear it regularly and reapply it often. But much better than lipstick are Neutrogena Lip Protectant and Chap Stick with sunscreen. These have the obvious extra advantage of having excellent sunscreens contained within their formulations. They're especially good if you're going to be out in the snow in the wintertime, because the cold, dry air and intense sun damage can destroy soft lips quickly. If you're not going to be outside much, regular Vaseline is an excellent product for restoring the necessary moisture to the lips. However, it's pretty easy to lick it off from time to time, so you'll have to concentrate on applying it frequently.

Will a humidifier help dry skin? Yes, low humidity should be corrected if at all possible. This can be done quite adequately by obtaining a good humidifier. The whole-house type, although more expensive, is the best because you can regulate your entire environment with the touch of a button. Such a humidifier will commonly be able to increase the humidity to 45 to 50 percent, which should be sufficient to help your dry skin, assuming you're following my advice on bathing, soaps, bath oils, and so forth.

Another way, of course, is to buy the single-room type of humidifier. Be sure not to get a dehumidifier, though. That could be disastrous. You might also consider leaving pans of water near heat duct openings, on radiators, and in other places. It even helps if you'll leave the commode lids open and leave a one-inch layer of water in the plugged bathtub all the time.

Another variant of dry eczema is called nummular eczema. Nummular eczema is dry, scaly skin with coin-shaped patches. It's the most common form of winter itch on the arms and legs. Though actually a type of xerosis, it can be somewhat harder to clear, and you may need lotions containing cortisone to get it under control.

The spots begin as tiny circular patches that are most often said, by the patients and some of their referring doctors, to be ringworm. Antifungal creams don't have much effect except to temporarily heal a patch or two, just because the medicine is slightly moisturizing.

IS DRY SKIN HEREDITARY?

You bet! But it's hard to tell a person if he or she will get it or pass it on, because so many of us have dry skin anyway. In general, light-skinned, fair-haired, blue-eyed folks are dry-skinned, and dark-complected people are less dry.

Many patients ask if it helps to eat oily foods to aid their dry skin problems. The oil a person eats is broken down into its component parts just like any other food we eat. It never reaches the skin as oil. So forget it.

Remember, if you take a few easy precautions against winter itch you can make dry, cold weather a lot more tolerable. Moisturize, lubricate, virtually lather on the lotions during cool, dry weather, or whenever you itch, scale, and flake. You'll feel "cutaneously comfortable" if you do!

$\mathscr{E}$czema

TREATING THAT AWFUL ITCH

One of my dermatology professors used to say that the itching of eczema was one of the most disagreeable sensations a human being could have. He had a neat trick for solving the scratching dilemma. After prescribing a medicated cream for patients (to cut down on inflammation), he advised them to put a little of the cream on the flat of the finger pad and to actually rub it into the itchy spot as many times a day as was needed. In this way he allowed the patients to do a "modified scratch" without injuring the skin. He also got the remarkable bonus of applying the topical cortisone cream in a very efficient manner, that is, rubbed well into the skin. This technique has worked so well for me during my years in practice that I use it for virtually every patient with an itching problem.

It's not hard to see from the description of the itch involved in eczema that it does no good whatsoever to admonish or scold a child for scratching. This only increases the guilt of the child and the guilt of the parents, who usually mistakenly assume that they have somehow given their child this disease through something they have done. Eczema is an unfortunate problem of children (and of some adults), and it would be unwise to punish our children or ourselves because of their misfortune in contracting this terrible disease.

Although some children do grow out of childhood eczema, the problem often evolves into a chronic smoldering eczema of the neck or hands as the patient ages. While cortisone creams can help the inflammation, it is often necessary, as I've suggested, to prescribe antibiotics because of the infection that occurs in eczema scratch marks. Don't worry too much if your doctor keeps your child on antibiotics for a significant length of time: very few cases of severe eczema will clear without them. Topical antibiotics (like the new Bactroban) can occasionally be of help, but you run some risk of sensitizing your child or making him or her allergic to the neomycin and other ingredients in these drugs. So if your doctor gives your child a topical antibiotic and if a worse rash develops instead of steadily clearing, the doctor should consider a possible allergic reaction to the topical antibiotic. I use topical antibiotics for my patients, but very selectively.

Sun, in general, does not help. A child with eczema needs moisture and general skin care to improve. The real reason why kids with eczema do better during the seasons of the year when the sun is brightest (spring and summer) is because of the increased humidity, not the sunlight. These children do not need the damaging rays of the sun.

Be sure to read the section in this book on Dry Skin (xerosis) for further advice on handling the skin of young eczema patients. This is vital to their skin health.

HOW TO PUT OUT THE FIRE
ON YOUR CHILD'S SKIN

Although it's possible to write an entire book on the subject of childhood eczema, I'll attempt to give you the salient features of the disease and the treatments that can help.

Common eczema of childhood is usually called atopic eczema. Atopic means "altered reactivity." This means that affected children have a family tendency to develop dry, itchy skin that scales and cracks. Often it forms large infected patches on the fronts of the elbows and the backs of the knees.

To illustrate how severe the problem can be, I would like to tell you about a five year old named Andy who was brought to me when I was a resident at the Medical College of Georgia. When I entered the room, all I could see was the blur of Andy's hands scratching his skin almost everywhere. Hardly a square inch of his body was spared from the torture of atopic eczema. Some areas were so bad that they were split open wide and literally dripping pus from scratch marks he had made. Andy's mother was in a real tizzy, scolding him almost constantly to stop scratching. She did not know that he was literally unable to stop scratching when his skin was that inflamed.

I questioned his mother about his problem, and it seems that he had trouble with itchy skin ever since infancy. At that time he had what they thought was a severe case of cradle cap that never cleared up. With time it had spread severely to the fronts of the arms, the backs of the knees, and the neck area. Most recently, during the Georgia summer heat, it had become infected, compounding the problem.

She told me that Andy's father had asthma and hay fever and that most of the family had severe sinus troubles. These are common associated findings in families of children with atopic eczema.

Further questioning revealed some reasons why Andy's eczema failed to clear up under the care of his pediatrician. His mother said that when Andy was an infant, the pediatrician had recommended a potent antibacterial soap. His mother thought that since this was recommended by his pediatrician it was a good treatment for atopic eczema. Actually, the soap had only irritated it. She had also been bathing him three times a day! No wonder the little tyke had skin as dry and cracked as the Mojave Desert! She had been washing out all of his natural skin oils for years.

I began a three-pronged attack to save poor Andy's skin. First, since all his scratch marks were badly infected, an internal antibiotic was absolutely required.

Second, since his main problem was skin dryness, I cut him down to one bath per week and changed him to Dove soap (other superfatted soaps are ok too) if he used any soap at all. Baby soap is okay, too, in moderation; but I see problems due to overuse of it in cases where it's assumed to be harmless. Some kids do even better by avoiding soap altogether and rubbing on a little Cetaphil lotion until a lather almost forms, then wiping it off with a tissue or towel, leaving most of this wonderful moisturizing lotion right on the skin.

Let me digress a minute to tell you a little story about a child who was treated by the renowned dermatologist Dr. J. Lamar Callaway at Duke University. One day he prescribed a "generic" cream for a child with eczema as bad as Andy's. The cream was in a large one-pound jar that he dispensed for a few cents to the family along with instructions to apply it thinly to eczema areas twice daily.

The child returned two weeks later with almost complete healing of his eczema, and Mom demanded, "What was in that 'mystery cream' of yours?"

"Just a little stuff we call 'Cream C' around here, that's all," he said.

"Cream C?" she asked, "What's the C stand for? I want to know what I'm putting on my child!"

"Well, if you must know," he said, "the C stands for plain, pure Crisco, right off the supermarket shelf!"

It's true! It works! It's probably one of the best and safest moisturizers ever found, although not very aesthetically acceptable. But Dr. Callaway had found, over the years, that mothers just wouldn't use the stuff if they knew it was Crisco, no matter how effective it was. That's why he started calling it Cream C.

Third, getting back to Andy, I started him on a hydrocortisone cream just strong enough to cool the fires of inflammation burning in his eczema.

These principles are very important in the treatment of your child. The fact is that Andy probably had atopic eczema because he had the wrong ancestors. The disease definitely is hereditary. We know that children of families having a lot of sinus trouble, allergies, hay fever, rhinitis, and hives have a greater incidence, or frequency, of atopic eczema.

The fact that eczema victims may have allergies of other types does not mean that an allergy causes the eczema. This skin disease seems to be completely independent of allergies that are usually treated with shots and desensitization. In atopic dermatitis these methods are of very little use.

The primary fact to be remembered in atopic dermatitis is that these kids itch, and so they will scratch. There is absolutely no use in telling a child with this problem not to scratch these spots. The disease itches so intensely that the child has little or no choice whether or not to react to the itching. The child actually scratches hard enough to scrape open the skin because the pain induced by scratching and tearing away at the skin is actually more tolerable than the itch itself!

$\mathcal{E}ye\ \mathcal{C}are$

INFECTIONS FROM COSMETICS

Several years ago researchers discovered that mascara (as well as other cosmetics) could become rancid with time. Bacteria were overgrowing in the cosmetics. Since this could possibly infect the eyes, users were warned to replace their mascara on a regular basis.

Eye infections did indeed begin to show up, and these were occasionally traced to a very bad practice at cosmetic counters. We've all seen demonstration cosmetics displayed in women's areas of department stores. These are being used by many different women, thus causing many possible strains of bacteria to collect in the demonstration unit. Ophthalmologists (physicians specializing in eye care) warned the public about the possible contamination and encouraged cosmetic companies to distribute individual, single-use packets of "tester" cosmetics. If the practice somehow reaches mascara, or if salespeople will just not permit the testing of mascara, the infection problem may be greatly lessened.

Eye infection is not the sole worry in regard to mascara. Leading dermatologists and eye care doctors specializing in cosmetic problems have warned that the mascara brushes themselves can cause damage and embed dangerous bacteria into the cornea (clear part of the eye), if the eye is touched. So the recommendation is that one should never touch the eyeball itself with any cosmetic applicator.

Women should never apply eye cosmetics in moving vehicles. One dermatologist recently remarked that she actually saw a woman at a stoplight drive away when the light changed, while simultaneously applying her mascara. (As yet no word has been received on whether she incurred any traffic injuries!)

A few years ago, and occasionally even now, a woman who is applying eye cosmetics to the lower lid margin, even inside the lashes, comes into my office with an eye irritation. Applying eyeliner to the extreme edge of the lid inside the lash line is the most dangerous of all eye cosmetic application techniques. At the moment the liner is being applied to the lid line, the brush is at its absolute closest to the eyeball. Also, the liner itself, if contaminated, has an excellent chance of getting into the eye directly. The look is alluring, but it may lure you into some very sight-threatening eye diseases.

DARK CIRCLES UNDER THE EYES

For years I didn't think dark circles under eyes really existed, or if they did exist, that they certainly wouldn't fluctuate with tiredness, and so on, the way people said they did. But then I heard an excellent professional talk by an allergist who had studied this condition extensively, and he had an interesting explanation for the darkness.

The eyes, and the bony orbits or sockets that hold them, have extensive blood circulation in and around them. On the upper cheeks and lower lids, these vessels form a plexus, or weblike network, just under the translucent skin. The skin is so thin in this area that they can actually be seen. As a person grows tired during a long day, or if he or she has sinusitis or allergies, the blood circulating through these vessels slows down and dilates the veins wide open. The bluish color shines through then, making what appears to be a "dark circle" under the eye.

There's no really good way to get rid of them, but they are not as likely to be prominent if you've had enough rest and if you don't have sinusitis or allergies. Cosmetics work wonders here.

YELLOW PATCHES ON THE LIDS (XANTHELASMA)

Yellow bumps and spots on the lids are quite common. These spots are called xanthelasma. This word is derived from a Greek word meaning "yellow plate," which is exactly what they look like. They represent a minor collection of oil below the surface of the eyelid skin. In some patients, they signify high levels of fats in the blood, such as cholesterol and/or triglycerides. In fact, we usually check patients for these abnormalities prior to treating them.

Xanthelasma lesions can be treated in many ways. It's the nature of these "oil slicks," as we call them, to recur, so don't be too surprised if they grow back after treatment.

Besides surgery, some dermatologists paint the spots with dilute trichloroacetic acid. This causes a scab to form over the spot, and over the next week or two the yellowish plaque dumps right out. Usually, this occurs without any scarring.

Electrosurgery, such as that used on the skin tags (small out-pouchings of otherwise normal skin), can also be used with great success. Just remember that with any method of removal, recurrence is the rule rather than the exception.

Fingernails

PROPER CARE OF OUR "FIRST TOOLS"

One cool summer morning, the first cave dweller was bitten by the first flea. The cave dweller instinctively scratched the itchy wound with a fingernail and unwittingly became the first human user of a tool in the world's history.

Actually, this story isn't as farfetched as it sounds, for our nails are truly responsible for our ability to manipulate fine objects. This function still persists, naturally—just watch someone trying to remove an adhesive bandage, or separate a sticky label from its backing, or perform any of a thousand other daily functions for which we use our nails, and you'll realize their importance.

But with civilization came another function of fingernails. They are now considered just as important for their decorative function. Everyone wants good-looking nails, and this section will tell you the up-to-date secrets to maintaining these important skin appendages in their best shape.

FINGERNAILS HAVE R-R-RIDGES

Fingernail ridges are a constant, but annoying problem, with a whole set of different causes. Chief among these is hand eczema, a scaly inflammation of the skin around the nails aggravated by excess water exposure and other factors. You see, the nails are made deep under the nail fold (cuticle) and then grow out slowly to appear as what we know as nail plate, the hard part of the nail. If any inflammation or irritation occurs around the nail fold area, it quite easily disturbs the growth pattern of the nail plate, producing a ridge.

The second leading cause of fingernail ridging is manipulation of the cuticle. Cuticle means "little skin," and as a tiny patch of normal skin, it takes care of itself completely, needing absolutely no help from us. Certainly, a small amount of skin temporarily hangs onto and drifts out onto the nail plate from time to time, but that was meant to be there as a protection for the delicate tissues below that are actively engaged in making the nail plate. Vigorous pushing back of the cuticles, therefore, will cause ridging in almost everyone.

Several years ago, a company was distributing a new nail product. They sent crews to the largest and best department stores in the land to give demonstrations. The product was basically an extremely refined polishing system designed to remove surface lines and ridges from the nails. It did this so well that customers did not even have to wear nail polish, and they still looked as if they were wearing an ultrasmooth coat of clear polish at the time.

Needless to say, I was impressed. My wife and I caught up with them one spring day in a department store in Atlanta and decided to try the stuff. She loved it and coaxed me into letting them try it on one of my nails, so that I could recommend it to my patients. When the demonstrator heard that, she was determined to give me a good impression of the system, so she really put some pressure into the polishing steps. There were several steps, and when she finished, my thumbnail shone like the sun! I was ecstatic that I had made this wonderful discovery and couldn't wait to get back to my home in Augusta to tell everyone what I had found. We were, of course, always looking for a magical way to smooth out rough nails for our patients with psoriasis, eczema, and fungus problems.

We residents were recommending the stuff almost daily for a couple of weeks, until I noticed something strange happening to my demonstration nail. I was growing a huge, deep ridge out from under my cuticle. Aghast, we all waited for our patients to come back with the same ridges, and sure enough, they began to complain of this over the next several weeks. They all grew out normal nails again, but we surely had a group of worried residents for a while.

So you can see the effects of any pushing or trauma on the cuticle area. Treat these tender areas gently, and they'll continue to make you a smooth nail plate. Vigorous pushing back of the cuticles can cause deep ridges in the nails. Cuticles are normal. Leave them alone. Vigorous buffing also ridges nails. Beware!

Psoriasis and other diseases, such as thyroid abnormalities, can also cause ridging of the nails. Your dermatologist can investigate these further. Sometimes if the underlying cause is corrected, the nails get better.

Ridges have many causes, but ridges on the toenails, and not simultaneously on the fingernails, suggest trauma as a main cause. That is, it's very possible that something you're doing to your toenails could be causing the ridges. How about tight footwear? That's one of the chief causes of the large toenail ridges. Are you in an occupation where things often drop on your feet? Have you had any injuries over the last few months that might be showing up now? Remember that toenails grow only about two millimeters per month, so an injury could be two months old or so before you'd even see it!

I remember dropping a table knife on my great toe about five years ago, and the ridge and bruise didn't grow out and show up for weeks. Try to search your memory for injuries; it may produce some satisfying results.

HAVE YOUR NAILS GONE SCHIZ?

Often, nails split back in layers. Often, as soon as they get past the end of the finger, they split. This problem is one we all have to some degree, called onychoschizia (splitting of the nails). It's perhaps the most common complaint we hear about nails. The causes are vague, to say the least. One of the world's leading nail experts, Dr. Nardo Zaias, says in his book, *The Nail in Health and Disease,* (SP Medical & Scientific Books, 1980), "This layering of the nail plate is not an uncommon abnormality. *Absolutely nothing is known about it!"* (Italics and exclamation, mine.)

In practice, however, there are some things that do seem to aggravate onychoschizia. My patients get worse with this condition when they are in water frequently. Also, as with other nail problems, using polish remover frequently worsens it. And I would certainly eliminate the moistening agent for a while to see if you get better. I also think most of my patients do better if they keep their nails polished all the time. Agents such as Hard as Nails may help, too. Try not to be too conscientious about removing all the polish for what could be just a minor touch-up.

There are a few other secrets you should know about keeping your nails in good shape. Throw away your nail clipper, and get a sharp new one every three months. Clip your nails only when they're wet (say, after a shower or bath). After you clip your nails, file them gently with a fresh emery board. Use a "down-and-away" motion from front to back on the nail edge.

And if you still have a problem with nail splitting, use a heavy moisturizer containing phospholipid, urea, or lactic acid to soften your nails. If you use such lotions frequently, you may not have further problems with splitting. We've all heard people say that eating gelatin can help this problem. Being a scientist, I cringe when I hear someone utter that dermatologic falsehood. It's equivalent to the tribe of headhunters who reportedly said that if you wanted to be as brave as someone else, you must eat his heart, and so forth. If you want to have the best fingernails, must you eat modified fingernails (gelatin is ground-up horses' hoofs)? How disgusting. And it doesn't work. The protein provided by gelatin is constantly made available to your nail-making apparatus anyway. So forget the gelatin. One nail expert thinks it may even do more good to soak your nails in gelatin than to drink the stuff.

And calcium to harden the nails is completely useless. Calcium is used to make bones and teeth hard as nails, not vice versa!

Occasionally, patients notice excess ridging of the nails when they wear artificial fingernails. Sometimes the glue that comes with the nails will not keep them on, so some people use Super Glue to keep them on at least a week. I've got one patient who went to a salon where they use cyanoacrylate. She has become so allergic to this substance that her nails look worse than ever, and the cracking and irritation get so bad sometimes that she needs to get oral cortisone to shut down this horrible process. Still, she persists in using the false nails occasionally. I guess she thinks that someday she'll lose her allergy to the glue, but that'll never happen.

NAIL DOTS AND WHITE LIES

Been telling white lies lately? That's where the little white dots in nails are supposed to come from, you know, at least according to the old wives' tale. Actually, they come from minor nicks and blows to the fingernails, causing a tiny dot of abnormal growth. So no matter what you take, you will still get these spots if your nails are hit from time to time. Zinc's useless for this purpose.

Realize that your nails are specialized organs of the skin. A little regular maintenance of these delicate, useful, and beautiful tools will keep them in shape for a lifetime.

Freckles

BANE OF THE BONNIE LASS

I've had many women (and occasionally men) patients who have complained vigorously about having had sun freckles produced on their skins through sun indiscretions in the past. Sun freckling is a problem many women (and men) face in their search for a tan. Even short, intense exposures to the sun can change the skin's texture and color forever.

Treatment? That all depends on how many freckles you have and upon the amount of pain you're willing to go through to have them removed. My patient Wanda had many of them.

"Help me get these nasty freckles off, Dr. Bark!" she exclaimed.

"I'd love to," I said, "but you know that involves freezing them all with liquid nitrogen?"

"Sure, go to it," she said. She slid out of her shirt, revealing a whole forest of brown freckles of every size and shape. She looked like a leopard!

"Uh, where would you like me to start freezing?"

"Gosh, I don't know," she said. "Maybe if you'd just get a fifty-five-gallon drum of the stuff, you could hold me by the heels and just dip me in!"

It would have been a mammoth job indeed. We decided to frost the biggest and most objectionable ones lightly, leaving her "adolescents" to grow up a little before we chilled them off. I'm sure she'll be back, on and off, for years because of her sun indiscretions.

SUN FRECKLES

Flat, usually nonscaly brown spots, often found on the sides of the face and elsewhere, are called actinic lentigo or sun freckles. Sometimes they have an element of actinic keratosis (see Skin Cancer section) in them. They are removed beautifully by light cryosurgery. They darken with continued sun exposure, so protect them from sunlight if at all possible.

88

Fungal Infections

A FUNGUS RUNNING AROUND IN CIRCLES

We've all heard of "ringworm" infections in kids. There's a lot of folklore about these rashes, too. First, there's no worm in ringworm. But the circular lesions, or spots, of this fungus certainly give one the impression that there might be. The term may have been around for over 500 years and was probably used to describe not only the ringlike lesions of skin fungus, but also psoriasis, eczema, syphilis, and many other diseases through the centuries.

Why does it spread in a circle? No one knows. It may very well have something to do with the immune system, but as yet we're not smart enough to figure it out. Maybe each individual cell the fungus attacks acquires immunity to it, allowing the fungus to spread in only one direction—outward. This results in the formation of a circle as it progresses.

We do know it's contagious, however. Ringworm of the scalp, for instance, used to be an almost occupational disease of moviegoers. The backs of old-time theater seats were chock full of the fungus, and many unlucky kids caught "the tetter*" from leaning their heads back to watch the show.

Treatment of tinea corporis (ringworm) relies on oral and topical anti-fungal preparations and the good news is that the time needed to resolve it is usually vastly less than other body fungi. Often a month of internal treatment will be enough. Obviously, there is no worm.

---

*From the Old English "teta" which meant any type of eczema or skin eruption.

TWO-FOOT-ONE-HAND DISEASE

I once talked to a fellow who had come home from Vietnam with a condition he would have preferred to leave behind. He had scaly skin and deformed nails on one hand and on both feet. The other hand was absolutely clear of scale or any problem. His description of the fungus could be right out of a textbook! We call this "two-foot-one-hand disease," or, in medical terms, tinea. It is the result of a stubborn fungus that, like long strands of vegetable matter, actually grows into the upper layers of skin, where it multiplies. Sometimes, it lasts for years and can affect the fingernails severely, causing them to be so thick that they are functionally unusable.

The great mystery is: Why does the fungus grow on only one hand? Frankly, we don't have the answer to what causes this strange condition. Researchers have tried to relate it to handedness, thinking that one hand would undergo different conditions than the other, but such theories appear to be invalid. Perhaps the immune system is responsible, but the answer is not yet in. Much more research is needed to adequately explain two-foot-one-hand disease.

The longest-lasting case I've ever seen was that of a forty-year-old farmer who showed up in my office a couple of years ago. He was explaining to me a problem of "diesel oil irritation" on his right hand. He had had it for twenty years! He showed me a fine, powdery scale on his right palm, which aroused my suspicion. When I asked him to show me his feet, both were covered with the classical thick scale of tinea pedis (foot fungus) infection.

Worst of all, the fingernails on the affected hand and most of his toenails were as thick as horses' hoofs. I told him what he had, but he insisted it was just diesel oil irritation, caused by a spill of fuel onto his hand long ago. So I did what's called a KOH preparation on the scaly material to demonstrate the fungus. When I looked into the microscope, the scale contained so much fungus that I thought it would reach out and grab me!

I told him the good news. An oral antifungal pill called griseofulvin could probably heal his hand and feet over a period of time. Hands usually take six months or so, but toenails and feet, much more difficult areas to clear, can take as long as one to one and a half years. It takes twelve to eighteen months to grow a new toenail, but only six to nine months to grow a new fingernail.

Over the next few months, his hand began to clear for what I'm sure must have been the first time in his adult life. He's about the most grateful patient I've ever seen! He never really thought he'd have a smooth hand again.

NAIL FUNGUS— HARD AS NAILS TO TREAT

Many people have fungus infections of the nails only. This scruffy buildup of dead material under the nails makes them look as if they are whitening and rotting right off the tip of the fingers. This is a difficult infection to treat topically, that is, without internally taken medicines. The nail is made of a waterproof protein called keratin, which is specially built to protect the end of the digit and to keep chemicals, including antifungals, out. That makes the job of the pharmacologist, or drug designer, doubly hard because, in a sense, the skin is working against its own cure.

The simple fact is that normal lotions that will kill a fungus in almost every other skin area will not touch those beneath the nail. That's why oral medicines, which get to the nail fungus from the inside, are needed. Over the last few years, a method has been developed for painless removal of diseased toenails. Called the beeswax-urea method, it was discovered in the former Soviet Union and was brought back to the United States by a prominent visiting dermatologist-professor. In our office we call it the "Russian formula" bandage.

The technique consists of the application of a paste made from beeswax and urea. These two ingredients soften the nail plate, but, remarkably, only where the plate has underlying disease, such as a fungus. The paste is plastered on the toenail, covered with a bandage, and left on for about seven to ten days. After this, the bandage and paste are removed, and all the diseased nail is then trimmed off—painlessly! Patients can hardly believe how well it works. Sometimes, if the whole nail is diseased, it will come off completely and painlessly, all the way back to the nail fold (cuticle).

When the nail is removed, we usually put the patients on oral and topical antifungals, so that their risk of regrowing a fungus-laden nail is greatly lessened. Special tricks, such as filing the thick nail flat with an emery board so that it's paper thin, can also help greatly as the nail begins to reemerge.

FUNGUS INFECTIONS OF FOOT SKIN

Some foot fungus infections begin as a blistering eruption or rash on the soles and insteps. A professor in my residency had a favorite saying: "A blister on the foot is fungus until proven otherwise." And he's absolutely right. Tiny, deep-seated blisters on the feet most often are fungus. It's really very easy to prove this when your doctor scrapes the top off one or more of the blisters. He or she can look at this material in the KOH preparation and confirm fungus in minutes.

UNDERARM FUNGUS—IT'S THE PITS!

Some men develop armpits that itch almost constantly. Though there are many causes of this, sometimes the armpit hairs are full of a yellow-gray coating that can't be removed. This can be a condition called trichomycosis axillaries. In this disease, bacteria adhere to the hairs but not to the skin. The hairs stick together and become a real nuisance. No one knows exactly why it strikes predominantly in the armpits. Of course, women who shave their underarms regularly don't have much problem with trichomycosis axillaries.

Treatment, as you may have guessed, is simple. Shave your underarms. If you don't like that prospect, you can get various topical antibiotics from your doctor or use a 1 percent formalin lotion, which can be made up by your pharmacist.

Hair

EITHER FAMINE OR FEAST

"Chrome dome," "baldy," "skin head!" We've all heard these terrible terms poking fun at men who have lost all or part of their hair. The use of such terms shows the almost universal importance of hair in our society as an indicator of virtually hundreds of different personality traits.

For instance, here are the results of a study published in the *St. Louis Globe Democrat:* Seventy-five percent of bald or balding executives surveyed agreed that their social life was affected by their hair loss. Ninety percent thought there was not enough research to find a cure, and a whopping 71 percent thought bald men were not as well accepted by society as those with hair.

Billions of dollars are spent on male and female hair care in our society each year. Hair is a vital component in the interaction between men and women. Whenever I have spoken before large groups, I've been deluged with hair questions. This section covers many different types of hair loss in some detail to tell the whole story of what we know and don't know about their causes and treatment. We'll discuss several experimental forms of treatment for hair loss. You should know about these treatments even if they're not yet FDA-approved or widely available in your area, so if they prove to greatly help hair loss, you'll already be familiar with them.

Beyond the investigational measures to solve hair loss, you should know about proper everyday hair care, especially if you're losing hair. And there are so many quacks and charlatans waiting to get their hands on your balding head; you must know how to avoid their clutches above all! So hang on to your hair as we discuss the many problems of hair loss and hair care.

MALE PATTERN BALDNESS

Ever since Hippocrates treated baldness with a sludge of opium, rose petals, and unripe olives, the treatment of baldness has been a major human concern. Many men feel that if they don't have hair, life is just not worth living. Some men, in fact, are those I call "wrappers." A wrapper lets one long clump of hair grow out of the horseshoe area of remaining hair so that he can wrap it around and around and around, spray it with hair spray or some other kind of glue, and partially cover his bald pate. I once knew a guy like this who would go out jogging in the wind, and at the end of running a single block would look like a shaved Cossack with a single, long, flowing scalp lock!

Other men calmly allow their baldness to progress and, I think, more or less feel it is a sign of virility more than anything else. It's hard to predict the way people will react to a problem that so obviously affects the way they greet the world and the way it greets them. But why do we lose hair? What can be done to hang on to what we have?

Male pattern baldness is called androgenetic alopecia (AGA). The term "androgenetic" tells a lot about the origin and expression of the condition. First of all, it is necessary to have the primary genetic material in order to go bald. That is, if you don't have the hair loss genes, you don't lose hair.

The genes, of course, are passed down through families by the male and the female members. It's a common fallacy that only the males in the family carry the gene, and that if your father had a full head of hair, you will automatically have one. But the gene does indeed pass on either side of the family; so it is necessary to search the family tree on both sides to find the link to the member with hair loss.

Besides the gene for baldness, it's also necessary to have the androgenic or male hormones required to activate the baldness gene. The situation may be likened to a lawnmower in a yard fall of grass. The grass cannot be cut (baldness) without three prerequisites. First, the lawnmower (the gene) has to be there. Second, gasoline (the androgenic hormone) has to be put in the lawnmower. Last, the engine cord must be pulled (age) to start the lawnmower.

The chief hormone I mentioned is called dihydrotestosterone (DHT). DHT is a very potent cause of "miniaturization" of the male hair follicle. Miniaturization? Yes, I mean exactly that; bald men are not bald at all. Their long, black, adult "terminal" hairs have just evolved into baby-fine "vellus" hairs, which are invisible, or nearly so, to the naked eye.

But the follicles themselves, which are the hair-producing units, are still intact. This leaves hope for future medicines that may be used to turn on those miniaturized hair follicles. We shall talk more about this later when we talk about treatment for male pattern hair loss.

Age is the final trigger for the onset of baldness. One of the many mysteries of baldness is why a young man of nineteen who has the same hormones and genes that he will have at forty-five often does not lose hair at the former age but will have lost perhaps much of it at the latter.

Dr. Norman Orentreich, the great hair expert and inventor of the hair transplant, likes to relate a story about identical twins, one of whom was castrated before puberty because of a testicular disease. His brother lost hair, but the castrated twin did not. At about age forty he received a series of shots containing male hormone. Six months later he was precisely as bald as his twin. He had needed the hormonal "key" to activate his hair loss.

VITAMINS

Vitamin deficiency does not cause hair loss except in the most dire circumstances. Many starving children of the world begin to lose their hair, which also undergoes color changes before the children die from malnutrition. It's nearly impossible to find that type of malnutrition on this continent. Of course, there are certain disease states, such as cancer and alcoholism, in which malnutrition can be this severe, but these are by far the exceptions. Don't waste your money on vitamin therapies. This includes all the special "hair vitamins" advertised in the lay press.

Many patients request information on wheat germ in regard to losing hair. Several world-famous hair experts have advised us dermatologists to have our patients avoid wheat germ in any form. I used a wheat germ shampoo myself for a year or two, because I liked its fragrance, but I too gave it up when I heard that wheat germ might possibly encourage hair loss.

The reason: The oil in wheat germ contains a male hormone-like substance which resembles that which causes AGA. Certainly it would be wise to avoid any possible source of such substances.

Patients who consult dermatologists about hair loss often complain about the ads in a men's magazine with questionnaires they are supposed to fill out and send in, so they can determine how to help with hair loss. Often they fire off a check, but don't get anything back! Why aren't people warned about this? Well, consider yourself warned. It's always been amazing to me how quick people are to fire off a check to a charlatan who has never seen them before. And often how reluctant they can be to visit a dermatologist with the necessary experience to properly evaluate their hair loss.

There are many magazine ads for "hair restorers." A patient once remarked in frustration, "If topical hair restorers worked, you'd have hairy fingers from applying them!" While this is an exaggeration, millions of balding males are victimized by baldness and hair-growth quackery each year. Most often the photographs and advertisements in men's magazines (and women's magazines, for that matter) are retouched photographs showing hair regrowth that cannot possibly occur with these methods. The other trick these charlatans use is to show a type of hair loss called alopecia areata, in which the hair regrows in almost everyone within six months. They pick a person with this disease in a spot where a person might ordinarily have male pattern hair loss, claim it is male pattern hair loss, and then show its "rapid regrowth."

Of course, all these products are worthless. There is only one certified agent currently available that will regrow hair in a person who has lost it due to androgenetic alopecia. More about it later. However, transplants can work wonders for the proper candidates.

TRANSPLANTS— WHAT YOU NEED TO KNOW

In AGA, hair can often be replaced by moving some of your hair to your less hairy spots. The transplant surgeon takes out small plugs of bald skin on the crown and replaces them with slightly larger plugs of good hair-bearing skin from the donor sites, usually at the sides of the scalp. (No, if you want curly hair, they will not take the donor plugs from your armpits!)

The surgery is usually bloody and very expensive. It can involve scarring, infection, and, rarely, rejection of the transplanted plugs. It cannot be overemphasized that you must have this done by a very qualified dermatologic surgeon or plastic surgeon. You must discuss predicted final results, progressive balding requiring further transplants, and all the complications involved.

Sometimes your plastic surgeon may want to do a "scalp reduction" operation before starting your transplant. In this procedure, some of the bald skin is cut away first, leaving a much smaller area to transplant later.

Why do transplant plugs continue to grow hair when they are put in a scalp that has lost its regular hair? There is some genetic component of remaining hairy scalp areas that keeps hairs growing even when transplanted to a new location. We don't know exactly what this factor is yet, but we do know that those hairs grow well, even when the surrounding skin has no obvious terminal hair growth.

The transplanted hairs will keep growing until exactly the same time that the donor areas begin to go bald. Luckily most people retain the hairs around the edge of the scalp for a considerably longer time. In fact, most rarely lose hair completely from these areas. Therefore, most hair transplantees will not have to worry about this problem, since their plugs are taken from areas that have good hair growth, and they probably will keep it.

Note that newer techniques called micrografts and minigrafts are now used to make the hairline virtually indistinguishable from a normal hairline. Most transplant surgeons are using these techniques.

You should also beware that there are many charlatans out there calling themselves "hair therapists," or "trichologists," and so forth, and who are not skilled at hair transplantation. If you would consider transplantation, ask your board-certified dermatologist for a referral to a transplant surgeon he or she would personally use, one who uses all the modalities available: scalp reduction, mini- and micrografts, and so forth. Never let anyone *implant* anything into your scalp. I have treated such patients who have had resultant scarring and disfigurement from such quacks anchoring hairpieces to the living scalp with sutures and other materials. Again, consider yourself forewarned!

HEADGEAR AND HAIR LOSS—A FREQUENTLY ASKED QUESTION

Many patients have requested info on losing hair because of wearing hats, football helmets, the ubiquitous baseball cap, and other headgear. Can these *cause* hair loss? Absolutely not! The number of old wives' tales (old husbands' tales in this case) concerning a cause for baldness exceed even the number of patients who are balding. Most of these inquiries are based on the theories that the blood flow under headwear is less, and this causes the hair to fall out. But circulation has very little to do with hair loss. It's not hard to prove this if one sees the tremendous bleeding that can occur with scalp lacerations. The scalp actually has the best circulation of any skin on the human body.

HAIR ANALYSIS

Hair analysis is an extremely sensitive testing technique for analyzing the chemicals of the hair, and it has been called nearly valueless by some of the world's leading hair experts. Of course it can tell you what's *in* your hair. The problem is that it also tells you what's *on* your hair! In other words we have so many pollutants, chemicals, and other matter in the air around us that these sensitive tests can be completely thrown off by the substances in the air around your hair. You could, for instance, live in downtown New York City and have a completely different hair analysis than does your identical twin who lives uptown. Also, the presence of cigarette smoke and other pollutants in our environment as well as hair creams, shampoos, and sprays makes these tests essentially useless. Only in a rare genetic malformation of the hair, with an absence of certain amino acids, can these tests be of any help.

Real hair experts do not perform many hair analyses. But the self-styled hair "experts" do, and they'll be very willing to sell you one of these tests in order to further the current holistic hype. Consult a real hair expert, your dermatologist, who has studied hair, its growth pattern, its makeup, and its diseases for years. You'll get straight information you can really use.

MASSAGES AND HAIR LOSS

Will massages help hair loss? Not in the least! The scalp circulation is already excellent, as I've mentioned, and massaging it will do nothing to help it further.

ROGAINE—
A NEW LIGHT FOR HAIR LOSS

This potent medication is used internally in very difficult cases of hypertension (high blood pressure), and was discovered to cause hair growth in areas that are not ordinarily covered with it. The medicine, when taken orally, is a very potent stimulator of dark, or terminal, hair growth, especially on the faces of females where, of course, it's usually neither found nor desired.

This discovery prompted the dermatologic community and the Upjohn Company, makers of the drug, to consider using this medication in the treatment of male pattern hair loss. But since there are many side effects to the medication when taken internally, it was necessary to plan an extraordinarily careful study to show any possible effectiveness of, and reaction to, the medicine. Rogaine produces noticeable regrowth of hair in about 30 percent of men under forty. In another 30 percent or so, the drug seems to help maintain the hair that the patient currently has. The remaining 30 to 40 percent of men have little or no regrowth.

It also seems important to start the medication as soon as possible after hair loss begins. The good news is that there are very few, if any, complications yet reported with the medication.

We don't yet know everything about how this medicine works. We know it is a vasodilator. This means that it opens up blood vessels quite wide and, through this mechanism, appears to reduce blood pressure when taken internally. It may be, therefore, that the effect of hair regrowth is produced by some action upon the blood vessels surrounding hairs. We know, however, that circulation is not the reason for baldness. Over thirty years of experience with hair transplants shows us that the donor site hairs will definitely live in areas of balding, so the circulation is fine in balding areas. Thus there must be something else to the action of minoxidil that we do not yet understand.

DAILY WASHING HELPS

It appears that the hormone DHT is secreted in the oil of the sebaceous (or oil) gland that attaches to every hair follicle in the scalp. Thus, the hormone lies on the surface skin and is therefore reabsorbed through the skin, thereby causing further loss when it reaches the hair follicle again. The "circulation" of this potent hair loss-causing hormone can be intercepted through a very simple technique—daily washing! That's right, daily washing can slow down male pattern hair loss! Use an excellent oil-removing shampoo such as Ionil, Neutrogena, or Ionil-T Plus on a daily basis. The hair should be lathered twice in order to ensure thorough oil removal.

"Age Thinning"

The hair loss that occurs in females in middle age and later is also a type of pattern hair loss. Sometimes it can occur in the male pattern on the crown, but more often it occurs along the lateral or side areas of the scalp, near the temples, and involves the receding hairline.

Females, of course, have a hormonal situation that resembles that of males, but it occurs later in life. The key is that at menopause the ovaries go into an inactive state and stop producing estrogen.

Rogaine is approved for use in women who are losing hair, too, but the earlier the problem is attacked with the medicine, the more hope there is of at least partially solving the ongoing problem of hair loss in women. It's been very adequately calculated that hair fall can consist of 100 or 125 hairs a day and still be normal.

Thin Hair in Children

I once had a grandmother complain, "My granddaughter has very thin hair. In fact, she is two and a half years old and does not have enough hair to even put a barrette in. Is she lacking something in her diet?" The fact that she doesn't have enough hair to put a barrette in may be because she has worn them in the past. Barrettes are an occasional cause of a problem we call traction alopecia. In this condition, the hair loss is due to chronic, slow pulling on the hair. Barrettes can do this!

As I've said previously, vitamins are not likely to be the problem unless the patient is on a starvation diet. I've seen several patients who have participated in weight loss programs (sometimes even those overseen by physicians) that have caused drastic amounts of hair loss.

The larger question for your granddaughter is, however, does she have a structural defect in her hair? There are several genetic conditions in which the hairs do not form correctly, having either weak spots or holes within the shaft, causing easy breakage. One of these peculiar diseases is called trichorrhexis nodosa. It is characterized by extremely frayed weak spots in the hair shafts that, under the microscope, look like two broomsticks shoved together. It's very easy to snap off the hairs at these weak spots. Your dermatologist can pull a few hairs and spot these strange disorders very quickly.

Treatment for this problem amounts to keeping a short hair style and avoiding manipulation whenever possible. Avoiding combing when wet will also reduce stresses on hair, and hair conditioners smooth the combing process.

Most people who have thin hair have a family tendency toward it and nothing can be done for this. As you can see, it's important to obtain the correct advice about how to manage easily damaged hair.

GRAY HAIR—SNOW ON THE ROOF

What to do about graying hair in men? Most consider it a "badge of honor" for surviving to their current age, but many want to remove all signs of gray. Grecian Formula is one way we've all heard about. It is a gradual coloring agent that contains the chemical lead acetate. The chemical attaches to the hairs and does not reflect light very well. This makes the hair surface take on a black look. For years dermatologists have okayed these products as long as the manufacturer's directions are followed. I personally like gray hair. Although Grecian Formula is probably safe to use, I would definitely follow the package directions very carefully and would be very careful to put it only on the hairs, and not on the skin. The real disadvantage is cosmetic—only various shadings of black can be produced, so men (or women, for that matter) with brown, red, or blond hair will find little use for the product.

Want a better idea? Why don't you try some of the new color rinses and dyes that are made "just for men"? Their safety records are good, and the color selection is almost infinite. Or better yet, have a professional salon help you mask your gray. So easy, and much faster results, too.

PROPER HAIR CARE

Hairbrushes are murder on your hair. The tension applied by the conventional hairbrush is so great that it can split, rip, and crack even the strongest of hair shafts.

Worse yet, combing hair when it's wet is about the worst experience ever for it. A Caucasian who combs the hair wet exerts terrific forces on it. Let it get at least partially dry before starting to comb. And be sure to use a wide-toothed comb.

The situation with blacks is the opposite. Blacks with curly hair should start combing gently with a wide-toothed comb when the hair is wet. The natural curliness allows it to spring apart so that the water acts more as a separator of the hair shafts and makes combing easier.

Hair shafts are inherently tough. They should withstand most forces in your daily life without having much splitting, fraying, or breakage. The old axiom, "Brush one hundred strokes every day," is as ridiculous as a mechanic who tells you to drive your car one hundred miles per hour eight hours per day in order to keep your tires in good shape. This folklore started when there were no conditioning shampoos or rinses. It was necessary then to comb out the natural scalp oil and spread it onto the hairs by frequent brushing. With today's modern shampoos and conditioners, this is no longer even the slightest problem.

And that's the take-home message: Use a conditioner. These agents drastically reduce the tension exerted on hairs by combing after washing. They coat and smooth the hairs with protein and other chemicals to keep them from tangling. Then combs glide across hairs smoothly, without exerting much force.

Something should be said about the frequency of your shampooing. Shampooing up to once a day does not cause increased hair loss or fracturing.

Hair dryers and manipulation are frequent causes of hair loss. I really don't mind hair dryers if they're used properly. By this I mean that a dryer should be used without an attached comb or brush. Did you ever think about how much your dryer weighs and how much more force it exerts than using just a simple wide-toothed comb? It's considerable! So use a blow dryer if you wish, preferably on the warm instead of the hot setting, and take off the attached comb or brush.

Of course, hot combs, hot rollers, and hot dryers are incredibly destructive to your hair. A hot comb can induce enough damage to completely fracture hairs, especially along the temple areas, where they're used most often.

PREGNANCY AND HAIR LOSS

There is only one type of hair loss dermatologists enjoy seeing in their offices. It is called "resting phase loss," or telogen effluvium. In order to understand this, it's necessary to know a bit about the way hairs grow normally.

The scalp hair cycle has three different stages. The first of these is the time of active growth called the *anagen* phase. This is the longest phase and can last several years for scalp hairs. During this time healthy follicles are taking in normal amounts of body nutrients and the cells of the follicle are cranking out large amounts of keratin, the special hair protein that makes up the shaft. It's really a time of remarkable activity in the microscopic factory we know as the hair follicle. But it can last only so long.

After four to seven years in most people, the scalp hairs cycle into a regression or involution stage called the *catagen* phase. During this stage, which lasts only a matter of days, the hair follicle shrivels at the end, signifying that its long anagen growth cycle is over. Growth stops quite abruptly now.

Following the catagen phase, the hair develops a bulbous enlargement at the end and is called a club hair. The club hair slowly splits off from the follicle. This *telogen* hair, as it's called, remains above the shriveled-up follicle for another month or two, until it is naturally sloughed out by pulling stresses on the outside hair such as wind and combing.

Resting hairs are the ones that come out when you pinch a bunch of hairs and very gently pull away from the scalp. The two or three hairs you obtain in this way were destined to fall out anyway, so don't think you've lost those hairs permanently. They're just cycling through their last phase before starting the new growth cycle.

After several months, telogen phase follicles cycle again into the growth, or anagen, phase.

The trick is understanding the type of hair loss you're having. Over 85 percent of the 100,000 hairs on your scalp are in the active growing phase during most of your life. Only a small amount, some 10 percent or so, are in the resting phase at any one time. In pregnancy, hormonal influences for growth apply not only to the enlarging fetus but also to a woman's own hair. It's locked into the anagen growth phase. This means that pregnant women often have long, luxurious locks growing by leaps and bounds. After delivery, however, the hormones normalize again and the hairs that were locked into the growth phase cycle simultaneously into the catagen and telogen phases. This means that a tremendous number of hairs are ready to fall out after their long stimulus to growth. And they do! Some women lose as much as 30 to 40 percent of their hairs during this period.

Here's the key. The hairs slowly regain their asynchronous cycling nature, which means that they begin to cycle independently of one another again. This means that almost every woman will get her hair back beautifully, as it was prior to her pregnancy, in just a few months. I know this is a little hard to believe when you're seeing handfuls of hair fall out after the birth of your baby, but it is true, and your dermatologist will reassure you of this fact. Stop worrying!

MISCELLANEOUS CAUSES OF HAIR LOSS

Hair Loss on the Pill

The birth control pill simulates the hormonal situation of pregnancy and therefore locks hairs into growth in most women. While it is true that some women lose hair from the pill, most actually have increased hair growth.

There are many endocrine gland problems that can cause hair loss. Certainly your dermatologist will want to know your menstrual history if you are losing hairs. He or she also will want to test you for the presence or absence of normal hormonal function in your ovaries, adrenals, and pituitary. All these glands are important in determining how much hair a woman has.

DRUGS

Many drugs can stimulate loss of hair when taken internally. Some high blood pressure medicines and other substances can cause this. Many cases have been reported, and you should ask the physician about your hair loss and possible drug-associated problems. Your physician may want to substitute another medication for a period of several months to see if your hair regrows. This process of elimination is often the only way to ascertain the real cause of hair loss.

SCALP ACNE

Acnelike bumps are often seen in the scalp. This is a typical acne eruption, unless some other cause is found. Inflammation of the follicle (hair-making unit) is occasionally caused by fungal and bacterial infection. This is called folliculitis. The control of folliculitis on the scalp is very difficult. You may need to be seeing a dermatologist regularly, but it's better than losing your hair with each of the bumps you get. Antibiotics and special treatment shampoos can usually control folliculitis quite nicely.

TREATING ALOPECIA AREATA (AREA BALDNESS)

Area, or spotty hair loss is called alopecia areata (AA). These well-delineated or "punched out" spots fall out in a matter of days for reasons that are incompletely understood. Studies of this disease indicate that it may be a type of autoimmune reaction; that is, the body is reacting defensively to its own skin and hair follicles, quite an unusual and rare situation.

Alopecia areata, or area baldness, is the kind of hair loss for which charlatans and hair treatment quacks used to demonstrate, in their "magnificent photographs," the apparently magical regrowth due to their usually harmless and always ineffective potions. But with this kind of loss the hair regrows on its own within six months. The natural pattern of AA is therefore one of healing.

The old-timers in dermatology used to think that AA was always related to emotions or a nervous condition, but that's probably doubtful. Although there are some well-documented cases of alopecia areata resulting from severe psychic trauma and mental upset, these are by far the exception rather than the rule. This is another case where physicians tend to attribute a disease entity to an emotional cause, when the real physiologic basis for the problem is unknown.

Treatment of alopecia areata is quite varied and depends upon the type you have. With isolated spots, it may be easy to get your hair back by having your dermatologist inject the spots with a dilute triamcinolone solution. This cortisone medication stays inside the skin, working to restore the hair for three to four weeks. In some cases, the injection functions as a permanent "cure," in that the hair does not fall out again. In other cases, it does fall out again, and new spots may even develop.

A slight hazard with the injection is that it can sometimes result in thinning of the skin and an irregular surface contour lasting for some months. However, the skin almost always returns to its original contour.

Other treatments work by inducing irritation on the scalp. One of the older remedies used by dermatologists is croton oil, a strong primary irritant that induces redness, inflammation, and soreness in the scalp. When this occurs, AA will sometimes resolve. Because of the extensive irritation, however, use of croton oil has been largely abandoned.

Other medications causing a healing irritation include anthralin, a plant derivative usually used in psoriasis to slow down the turnover of the epidermis. In alopecia areata it is used to cause irritation of the type that croton oil causes, but in a much more controlled fashion. It is not completely effective, though a significant percentage of patients will regrow their hair. Here again the irritation is the most important factor. If your scalp doesn't get irritated, you will not regrow hair. Even if it does get irritated, the regrowth process can take many months.

Recently, immunotherapy for alopecia areata has been developed. This investigational treatment involves the application of a chemical to which one can really get allergic, such as squaric acid. Such a chemical is first applied once to the skin under a patch test, to induce allergy, and then a lower concentration is applied to the scalp. Redness, swelling, and sometimes even blisters result. The goal is to cause a little mild redness and keep it there chronically.

The principle appears to be nearly the same as the "primary irritation" produced by croton oil and anthralin. Researchers think that the effectiveness of immunotherapy depends upon the calling up of the body's own lymphocytes, or defense cells, which actually suppress the allergy. It seems to be a case of one immune or allergic reaction canceling out the disease. It's a miserably itchy treatment, but it sometimes works to regrow hair.

In short, we don't know exactly how this all comes about, but research is under way to get the safest possible allergen that causes the least reaction and still grows hair. Over the next few years we should see great advances in this particular form of therapy for AA.

Another treatment for AA is called PUVA. While we'll discuss this new development elsewhere, mainly in regard to psoriasis, you should know that in some AA patients PUVA has restored hair dramatically.

The PUVA treatment involves taking an oral medicine called Oxsoralen, which makes the skin tremendously sensitive to the sun. In fact, it binds to the skin cell DNA (the actual molecules that control how the skin grows), causing damage to cell growth mechanisms. Two hours after the medicine is taken, the patient is exposed to long-wave ultraviolet light (UVA). PUVA is thus named from the Psoralen and the UVA.

If you want to know more about PUVA and its use in AA, talk to a dermatologist. There are complications with this therapy that you need to understand before undertaking it. Recently, many of these complications have been circumvented by the initiation of treatment with topically applied psoralens, instead of the internally taken type.

Last, with regard to alopecia areata, Rogaine applications may slow down the process or make the hair regrow. Each patient seemed to have different results with this medicine. In cases where the scalp hair is being lost extensively, we have had extreme trouble getting the hair back safely. While it is almost always possible to get hair to regrow with high to moderate doses of cortisone taken internally, this medication itself has extensive side effects when taken on a long-term basis. Therefore, no one relishes the prospect of putting a patient on an internal cortisone medication that he or she might have to stay on for years.

I do not approach internal cortisone treatment lightly, and neither should you. When injected locally into the spots of AA it's certainly safe, and very little absorption occurs to change other body systems. However, when cortisone is given internally in fairly high doses, as needed to regrow hair, such complications as salt and fluid retention, bone reabsorption, cataracts, ulcers, and psychosis can—and have—occurred.

In difficult cases, the most logical thing to do would be to go to one of the larger medical centers in which some of the newer investigative therapies I have described, such as DNCB and PUVA, are being used.

In most cases of extensive AA, called alopecia totalis, almost all the hair has gone from the head area. With some patients, every hair on the body falls out, a condition called alopecia universalis. These two conditions are occasionally associated with internal problems, such as anemias and thyroid difficulties, so any possible abnormalities in these areas should be checked. .

In the meantime, patients should realize they are not the only ones with this condition. There are hundreds of patients who are struggling every day with alopecia areata. Recently, the National Alopecia Areata Foundation (NAAF) has been formed to help such victims. You may write to them at:

National Alopecia Areata Foundation
710 C Street
Suite 11
San Rafael, CA 94910

The NAAF will be glad to keep you posted on new developments in treatment, as well as offer advice on ways patients and their families can cope.

TOO MUCH HAIR

What can you do if you have too much hair on your face? Well, though not a problem for men, naturally, women with a genetic history of hairiness in the family often notice an increase in the numbers and coarseness of facial hair around menopause or with surgical menopause (removal of the ovaries for a medical condition). Several drugs taken orally may help this condition.

Spironolactone is a potent diuretic (water pill) used in conditions such as fluid retention and high blood pressure. It causes potassium retention and therefore should not be used without follow-up by a dermatologist and/or an internal medicine specialist.

Other drugs for reducing facial hair include a fairly new one used mainly for the treatment of ulcer disease: cimetidine (Tagamet). It was noted that certain estrogenic effects took place with cimetidine, such as a slight increase in breast growth in men taking high doses. It then was theorized that it could reduce facial hair growth in women. This appears to have been the case. After eight or nine months, most female patients notice a decrease in the amount of facial hair, though not complete obliteration of it.

The problem with cimetidine is that it is very expensive, and the drug needs to be continued for a long time before any effect is seen. Why? Remember those three cycles of head hair growth? Facial hairs cycle in an eight- to ten-month anagen-catagen-telogen phase. This means that any effect will not be seen until the hairs normally fall out, usually some time after that eight- to ten-month time period.

This is a case in which a drug (Tagamet) is not yet FDA-approved for correcting hair loss. In a small number of patients, side effects have included mild and transient diarrhea, dizziness, somnolence, rash, headache, and rare cases of fever.

Experts in dermatologic hair care indicate that chronic epilation (pulling out hairs) may result in a permanent decrease in the number of hairs. That is, if hairs are waxed or tweezed time and again, numbers of them actually do not grow back. So women with this problem have several options. They can tweeze and wax, which actually is a very effective way of hair removal (albeit sometimes quite painful). They can bleach the hairs so that they are less noticeable, which has worked well for thousands of women. (This is best done with commercially available hair bleach. It's usually not irritating, if you carefully follow the instructions on the type you purchase.)

Electrolysis is the least desirable way to remove hairs. I've seen complications all too frequently from electrolysis, such as scarring and infection. Besides these problems, electrolysis really doesn't work as it's supposed to. Only a small fraction of the hairs are actually destroyed, and aberrant hairs can result if only part of the follicle is burned. These hairs grow crookedly into the surrounding skin, instead of out of the follicle opening, and severe inflammation can result. Home electrolysis machines not only are unsafe, but they're not very effective. It's nearly impossible to guide one of these instruments down the hair shaft the required distance to the hair bulb and burn out the hair bulb accurately.

Chemical hair removal? Works fine for some women! Nudit, Nair, Neet, and other barium sulfide-type agents can work. Magic Shave and Surgex are okay, but if your skin becomes irritated by such agents they should be discontinued. These last two are much more irritating, but can be tried on an isolated patch to test for irritation first, and then used. Beware not to use topical depilatories if you are using Retin-A for photoaging (age changes due to sunlight) or acne! It can cause much more irritation.

It usually is wise to use any depilatory only every third day or so, depending on tolerance. Hair removal creams do not remove the hair for good. Hair removal creams remove the hair at the surface or just barely below it and are very satisfactory for those who are not irritated by them. Bleach changes only the color of the hair and not its character or length. You can buy these concoctions in drugstores or the cosmetic sections of most department stores. Pulling hairs does not cause them to become darker or coarser when they grow back in.

One can even shave the face, and it won't change the character of the hair. I know that almost every woman reading this will think I'm crazy, but the facts are the facts. After all, how in the world could shaving off the top of a hair change the way the hair grows some two millimeters below the surface? If it did coarsen hair, bald men would shave their heads each morning to induce it to grow thicker.

As you can see, every person on earth is concerned about having or not having hair. It has become, and understandably so, a crucial part of our everyday lives. And yearly, we spend billions of dollars caring for our "strands of dead protein."

Hand Eczema

A FISTFUL OF PROBLEMS

Scaly, split, bleeding, dry hands . . . oh, the pain of hand eczema! Millions of men and women know the trouble it can cause.

Eczema means red, scaly, easily irritated skin. We don't know the exact cause, but we do know it's not contagious. It does, however, run in families.

In certain cases, eczema is a skin allergic reaction. Sometimes this can be tracked down with extensive patch testing, which will show contact allergy to one or more chemicals. These tests are done by applying the actual chemicals to the skin of the upper back. Occlusive patches and tape are used to maximize penetration so that they are more available to your immune system: The skin's reactions can be thus discovered more easily.

The patches are applied on one day and are read two days later for signs of itching, redness, swelling, bumps, and blisters. The angrier the reaction, the more significant the test result. I've had several cashiers, for instance, who were quite violently allergic to nickel, and handling coins was causing their hand problem.

I encourage patients with hand eczema to bring in everything they've used on their skin, including lotions, cosmetics, cleaning agents, detergents, soaps, perfumes, and shampoos. Many patients with hand and arm eczema turn out to be violently allergic to their shampoos.

While we don't currently know the exact cause of hand eczema, we do know many of the aggravants. Hand eczema occurs much more frequently in housewives, bartenders, cocktail waitresses, assembly line workers, and others who have their hands frequently immersed in water.

Even though hand eczema is sometimes called dyshidrosis, which means "painful sweating," it has nothing at all to do with the sweat glands of the hands. The old-timers used to think that the tiny, deep-seated blisters under the hand skin were sweat glands "welling up with disease," but thorough biopsies have shown these to be completely unrelated to the sweat glands themselves. Dyshidrosis of the feet also frequently occurs.

Because of the bad drying effects of water on the hands, keep your hands out of water whenever possible.

GLOVES TO THE RESCUE

How can you keep your hands dry when you must bathe your children, wash dishes, and do other household tasks? The best way is to buy three or four pairs of Dermal gloves and use these thin cotton gloves as liners under your regular rubber gloves. The reason for this is to always have a dry surface next to your hands. When one set of liners gets moist, either from splashing water into your gloves or from sweating, change liners. In this way, you'll keep a dry surface next to your sensitive hands all the time. If you can't get them at your local pharmacy, the address for the Dermal gloves is:

George Glove Company, Inc.
266 South Dean Street
Englewood, NJ 07631-5209

The next most common aggravant to hand eczema is soap. Try to avoid the antibacterial deodorant soaps. In general, they're too drying for hands that tend to get hand eczema. Also, those new liquid soaps in the sink-side dispensers are horribly drying. I suggest you use Dove Unscented, since it has been found to be the mildest soap. What about baby soap? It is a mild soap, but because it is assumed to be so much milder than other soaps, my patients tend to get into trouble with it because they use too much of it and because they use it too frequently. Stick with Dove—no one's ever found one milder.

Still, though, the best soap is the one that is never used! In fact, many dermatologists suggest that their patients with eczematous hands use only three to five drops of Cetaphil lotion because of its tremendous mildness. The lotion is applied, rubbed into a lather to cleanse the hands, and wiped off with a tissue, so that absolutely no water (other than that contained in the Cetaphil) ever touches the skin in the washing process.

Don't forget to rinse your hands well after each soap and water wash (if you absolutely must wash), and immediately thereafter apply a good moisturizing lotion such as Moisturel, Aveeno, Eucerin, or Purpose. These lotions allow you to maintain moisture in the skin of your hands by reapplying the natural skin oil you just removed.

While it goes without saying that harsh, irritating chemicals, such as solvents, turpentine, cutting oils, and detergents, should be kept miles from your delicate hands, you should know that vegetable juices like potato juice and onion juice will also greatly aggravate your hands.

For the present, there's no cure for hand eczema, but by following my advice you can keep your hands in the best shape possible at almost all times.

Once again, at the risk of breaking the bubble of those I prefer to call "psychodermatologists," I'll state that nerves don't affect hand eczema one bit. Jerry, a lawyer friend of mine, has horrible hand eczema, even at some of the calmest times in his life. At other, more stressful times, of which he has plenty, Jerry gets no worse. So I've never been a very staunch believer in the mind's control over the skin. Altogether too many physicians are, however, and I think that's unfortunate for patients.

One of my patients remarked that she got a burning reaction on her hands from handling a lot of our "central Kentucky favorite," hot banana peppers, deep fried right from her garden. This type of reaction is really not an allergy, but something called a primary irritant reaction. In an actual allergy, the rash is produced by the workings of a complicated system of immune factors inside the body. It would not happen to everybody who contacted the substance, just those whose immune systems were competent enough to recognize the substance as foreign.

However, in a primary irritant reaction, such as my patient gets from those wonderful peppers, everyone would get the reaction by handling enough of the offending substance. The cure is either not to handle them or else to wear rubber gloves when you do.

There is one exception to this situation that may have to be investigated for you by an allergist or a dermatologist. This is when contact with the peppers or other substances or certain chemicals causes a hivelike reaction. This is called contact urticaria syndrome and can be quite severe, even life-threatening. So if your hands swell and get very red on immediate contact with the peppers, see your physician right away. Incidentally, contact urticaria syndrome can happen with some of the oddest substances. One report concerned a little girl who swelled up every time her dog licked her. The dog's saliva activated the hivelike reaction.

Often, patients with hand eczema have a lot of cracking and bleeding around the fingernails. This is usually a variant of hand eczema that has occurred primarily in this location, rather than on the open skin of the hands. Some get the reaction mainly in the paronychial areas (the areas around the nail).

There are some other things to consider with the scaly paronychial areas, however. Women who use a lot of nail polish often dry out the skin around their nails by using too much acetone nail polish remover. I advise them to leave their polish on as long as they can, or to completely stop using polish for a while. This, plus a routine of heavy moisturization with a cream like Complex 15, should help tremendously.

Herpes

THE NEW LEPROSY

A man walked up to a waiter and asked, "May I please trouble you for a glass of water, sir?"

A woman behind a table, usually of good nature, glanced at the horrible weeping sores on his face and exclaimed, "Don't serve his kind anything! We don't want them around here!"

What a terrible disease leprosy can be! But wait. Not leprosy, you say? Of course not. It's a modern scene in any singles bar in our land. And unfortunately, it happens not once, but thousands of times daily to the unfortunate victims of the herpes simplex virus (HSV).

But why? Why, in this land of modern medical miracles of every imaginable sort, are we completely unable to shut off this terrible disease? Is there nothing we can do? Must we suffer this malady forever?

In this section, I'd like to examine the myths and madness surrounding the herpes controversy, from the standpoint of one who treats patients with HSV every day. I'll try to answer the common and uncommon questions about the disease and tell you exactly how I treat herpes of various types for my own patients, right in my office.

First, I should mention that for all the television shows, specials, and guest appearances I've done on the subject of HSV, I've gotten remarkably little mail asking questions about it. I've tried to imagine why this might be. At first I thought that the public was fed up with hearing about this incurable disease. But whenever we do a television show in the "call-in" format, the switchboards are swamped with calls. That led me to the real understanding of why more questions about the HSV aren't asked. Actually, *Time* magazine tipped me off to the possible solution with their detailed, excellent cover story on the national disaster of HSV.

The August 2, 1982, edition of Time stated, in an aside to the cover story, that they had a devil of a time finding models to pose for the front cover. This normally quite lucrative assignment went begging for models willing to be identified with the "scourge" of HSV. In short, people don't want to be identified in any way, shape, or form with the thought that they might have the dreaded disease. Even patients who are forced by the condition to seek treatment at my office are extremely reluctant to discuss their real problem.

Psychiatrists tell me that they're often consulted by patients who found it impossible to relate normally after contracting herpes. They say the victims feel "unclean" and "untouchable," just like the lepers of ancient times. But just as today's victims of true leprosy live in fair comfort in society, it's possible for the herpes patient to make his or her way successfully through social situations. Note that I didn't say easy, just possible.

Since there are two common presentations of herpes simplex, I've chosen to talk about the most common form, oral herpes, first.

COLD SORES

Oral herpes simplex is also known as fever blisters, cold sores, and "sun poisoning." Actually, that tells you a lot about what activates them. But where'd you get them in the first place, and why do they keep coming back? To understand your enemy may not, in this case, be to conquer, but it'll sure help.

The herpes virus is the ultimate parasite. It's a tiny DNA virus; that is, it has the very stuff of life, DNA, as its core. The virus probably hits us all at one time or another, but some of us are infected and some are not. Why? Unhappily, that's one of the numerous less-than-well-understood facts about this incredible organism. Some think since the virus lives inside the cell, the normal antibodies that defend us in similar situations cannot reach the virus inside the cell to kill it.

But which cells does the virus ordinarily live in? It actually maintains its home in the ganglia, or nerve clusters that emanate from the spinal cord and brain. So it's a nerve-infecting virus. To reinfect the skin with a new set of blisters, it must travel down the skin nerves and out onto the skin, where it again invades the cells of the skin itself.

There the virus activates and starts to reproduce its genetic material, thus making new virus particles. When this happens, the cells that had been previously infected with the herpes virus are burst open, or lysed, killing them and releasing thousands of virus particles into the surrounding area. It's during this time that the virus (and the rash it obviously causes) is spread to adjacent cells.

Once the new cells are parasitized by the virus, the whole process starts again. In this way, infection with the virus is perpetuated infection after painful, irritated, blistering infection. This very complicated replication process is one of the main areas in which research is being conducted to find a cure for herpes.

So sunlight activates your herpes sores? Join the club. It's probably the infection's most common aggravant. My office floods with herpes patients after every sunny, home football game at the University of Kentucky here in Lexington. Why it happens is not clear, but it appears that the damaging rays of the sun, which we dermatologists decry so often, stun the defenses of the skin cells in which the virus lives, thus allowing the virus to begin to multiply. The same mechanism is obviously at work for febrile illnesses (those with fevers) and, so the majority of dermatologists feel, in times of great emotional stress. Although those of us who consider ourselves "scientific dermatologists" like to think that no skin diseases are caused by emotions, it's really hard to stick to that opinion when patient after patient says that emotions bring on the attacks.

Vitamin B is completely worthless for fighting fever blister attacks. Its use is just another example of how lay people, when they don't know what to do for a skin disease, turn to the only thing they can control, diet and vitamins. Don't waste your time. Sunscreens are another story, however. They help by shielding the delicate skin cells from the sun's radiation. Without sun, the virus is not encouraged to multiply. Good sunscreens for this purpose include heavy opaque lipsticks, Chap Stick Sunblock 15 Lip Balm, and Neutrogena Lip Protectant.

Don't forget the age-old trick of wearing a broad-brimmed hat while you're outside. And try, if you can, to sit on the shady side of the stadium, or in a seat in partial shade anywhere.

What do we dermatologists tell patients when they ask where they got herpes simplex on their lips? Usually, as an infant, some careless, unknowing adult with a big, juicy herpes simplex sore on his or her lips scooped the child up off the floor and planted a huge, wet, virus-laden smooch right on the lips exactly in the place where the lesions are now. Disgusting! But it's a good lesson for all of us to remember—if you've got oral herpes simplex sores, you've absolutely no place around babies, infants, toddlers, or anybody else who doesn't especially want a lifetime of painful, weeping, oozing lip sores.

What's the difference between a cold sore and a fever blister? Each name just tells you the possible activator of the disease in an individual case. Colds, fever, stress, sunlight, and extreme fatigue are said to be initiators of the blisters.

GENITAL HSV

The herpes simplex viruses are generally divided into type I and type II. Type I was generally felt to be the type that attacked the lips, and type II was supposed to be the type that struck the genitalia. This division is a lot less useful today, because both types are found in both regions. This is thought to be a result of the changing sexual mores in this country, which permit orogenital sexual contact. This form of sex is directly responsible for the transference of the virus to the "new" areas where it had not previously been a frequent resident. It's a tougher virus and doesn't respond very well to the soothing treatments we usually use in the disease. We'll talk a lot more about treatment in a minute.

HERPES VS. GENITAL WARTS

Occasionally a patient will ask the difference between herpes and warts. Although they are both viral in origin, herpes is a blistering disease, first, last, and in between. It may ulcerate, or break down to weeping sores from time to time, but look like warts it doesn't. Warts are warts; herpes is herpes. But remember that they can both be considered to be venereal diseases, and they're both very communicable, so get yourself treated.

Some patients have a fever about twelve hours before they show up with HSV. Then tingling spots break out shortly in blisters.

What about this fever? We call this the viral prodrome, or warning signal that a new attack is coming. Many patients feel peculiar prior to the onset of the skin lesions and can very accurately predict that they'll have a new crop of painful blisters in a day or two. Maybe it's the fever that tips them off. I don't know of any good studies to show what causes them to know that they'll break out, but many do. Of course, the first-time victim often has a much more severe course than the patient with a subsequent attack.

HERPES AND CHILDBIRTH

Certainly the strain of a difficult delivery can result in the activation of a new crop of herpes blisters. Certainly herpes is a contagious disease and therefore can be transmitted. But there is little or no chance that other family members could get the disease from the delivering mother. In order to do this, it would be necessary to touch the spot where the disease occurs, or she would have to touch the spot and then immediately touch another person with some of the wet exudate (fluid from the blisters) on her hands. Both these possibilities would have to be considered unlikely if the barest minimum of precautions are taken, such as simple hand washing. In short, the family need not worry. But you should become acquainted with some of the other reasons why people get the disease on their buttocks.

In the *Schoch Letter,* a respected monthly newsletter circulated to every dermatologist in the country, a couple of explanations were proposed for why women contract buttock herpes. One of these is that they sit down on strange toilet seats (aren't they all?) from time to time, thus picking up the virus on a very logical part of their anatomy that contacts the seat. It is thought that the virus does actually live a short time on the seat after it has been deposited and infects its new host with great relish. At some time in the near future, then, the newly infected woman sits down with an active sore on her buttock, and unwittingly adds another statistic to the crowded rolls of herpes sufferers.

The other proposed explanation is, in my mind, even more plausible. It's called "spooning." After a man and woman complete sexual intercourse, the woman, because of her usually somewhat smaller stature, often rolls over with her back toward her mate, and he cuddles close to her, facing her backside. It's like two "spoons" fitting into one another. If he has a herpes sore on his penis, he drips virus onto her buttock for some time thereafter. Voila! A new herpes patient. It's a sad but highly probable explanation for this type of herpes in women.

ROLE OF TRAUMA IN HSV

I'm convinced that trauma plays a larger role in the development of herpes than previously thought. I have one patient, a notable athlete, who never had herpes prior to irritating his rear and sacral area doing strenuous sit-ups in a strange motel. Because he was anxious to stay in peak condition, he had done a tremendous number of sit-ups in nothing but an athletic supporter! The long "shag" carpet in the motel must have eroded away the protective dead layer of the skin just enough to embed the virus and start his lifetime infection with herpes simplex.

Also, some lipbiters tend to get recurrent HSV in locations where the superficial skin is removed.

ZOVIRAX—A VERY CLEVER DRUG

You should know about a new antiviral substance for herpes, called acyclovir (brand name Zovirax). Invented by researchers at the Burroughs Wellcome Company, it is one of the cleverest drugs ever devised. This substance kills the virus, but only after the virus itself activates the drug. They've actually enlisted the infection to help kill itself off!

In primary herpes simplex sufferers, the drug lessens symptoms, shortens the time of viral shedding, and promotes healing. The capsules are taken three times daily (400 mg.) at the first sign of an attack. They have several advantages. First, the capsules do appear to shorten the morbidity (pain and associated symptoms) and time course of the infection. The virus cannot usually be cultured from the lesions after taking the medicine for only twenty-four hours.

Currently the medicine is FDA-approved for use in genital herpes simplex. It may also be used as a preventive, in doses of three

200 mg. capsules daily, for up to twelve months. Again, this medicine is not a cure, but it's by far the best drug ever developed for HSV.

An intravenous form already on the market apparently helps those who develop generalized herpes simplex. This disease usually afflicts patients who are very ill due to some other serious cause, such as lymphoma or other types of cancer, or else immunosuppressed because of a transplant of some kind.

Another problem with acyclovir is the development of resistance to it by the virus. This could be a very drastic consequence: Since the virus is "smart" enough to skirt the drug (as some variants of herpes simplex do with acyclovir), this may severely limit the drug's usefulness in the treatment of common herpes simplex.

Until the cures for the viral venereal diseases such as herpes simplex are found, sexual relationships must be handled the same way porcupines make love—very carefully. Get to know your prospective partner. Don't bed down with anyone who appears to be in pain or who has sores of any kind anywhere. Do not have oral sex with anyone who has lip sores, swellings, or fever blisters. Ask your prospective partner if he or she has any communicable diseases such as AIDS, herpes, gonorrhea, syphilis, warts, or molluscum. Certainly not everyone is completely honest, but believe it or not, some still are. And use condoms; they may protect you from not only the herpes infection but also from many other venereal diseases.

Not long ago, I saw a personal ad for a person with herpes looking to date another who also had the disease. Sounds like a bright idea, doesn't it, until you realize that you could be contracting another strain of HSV or getting it in an area where you never had it before. It's a terrible situation our sex-oriented society is in. The search goes on each day for a new compound that will finally put to rest the "new leprosy," but it hasn't yet been found. Perhaps chemists, vaccine researchers, and dermatologists will find ways to prevent the spread of HSV in the near future, but for now, limiting contacts, investigating them, and frank discussion of sexually transmitted diseases are the only ways available to someone trying to live a disease-free existence.

Recent studies show that the HSV can be cultured from the skin even when the actual sores are not present. This makes the "swinging single" life even more complicated. The bottom line appears to be: Do your thing, if you must, but do it carefully and with your eyes wide open to the possible consequences.

SHINGLES—A HERPES VIRUS

The virus that starts shingles actually is one of the herpes viruses. But it's only phylogenetically related to herpes simplex. That is, you don't catch shingles from sexual activity or herpes simplex from a shingles patient. Just thought I'd clear that up before we start to talk about shingles.

The virus that causes shingles is called the varicella-zoster virus (VZV). All of you who are parents and who have seen your children through all the typical childhood diseases probably recognize varicella as chicken pox. Yep! That's right, chicken pox is the cause of shingles. Let me explain. Most of us have chicken pox as kids, it heals fine, and we think the disease is gone. But the virus actually goes into hiding in the nerve roots of the spinal cord, where it'll stay for the rest of our lives.

Later, VZV can be reactivated, only this time it doesn't produce a generalized case of chicken pox. Instead, a localized case of chicken poxlike blisters results from the virus invading the exact skin supplied by the nerve roots where it has hidden all these years. When the virus reaches the skin again, it starts to form blisters that are much worse than the childhood chicken pox.

Unlike chicken pox, shingles is a very painful disease and usually affects adults middle-aged and older. I've often been called to the cardiac intensive care unit to see patients with chest pain and a strange rash. The severe chest pain frequently started several days earlier than the rash, causing the physician to suspect a serious heart attack. Naturally, we're always happy to see a one-sided stripe of blisters appear on the patient's chest, indicating that he or she hasn't really had a heart attack at all.

Amazingly, you are contagious while you have shingles—not for shingles, but for chicken pox. A shingles patient never gives another person shingles, just chicken pox. So if you don't want members of your household to get chicken pox, then stay away from them when you have shingles.

It's been shown and remarked about for years that those with an atypical course of zoster, such as spreading of the rash outside the usual band-like area, are at some increased risk for cancer, usually of the digestive tract or lymph system. Remember the story of Paul in the introduction? It's in cases like these that we thank VZV for alerting us to such a problem.

How often is internal cancer related to shingles? It happens very rarely. In fact, some studies refute the claim that there's an association, but who could afford not to look? I personally study every VZV patient over forty-five. Usually, that amounts to getting at least a chest X-ray and a blood count.

You know how infrequently chicken pox makes scars? Well, when a patient gets VZV, in most cases he or she already has immunity to the virus. That's apparently why it just stays in one dermatome, or skin stripe. But the fact that immunity is present means that the reinfection is fought much harder by the body, resulting in a deeper mark in the spots where the blisters were. Most people who have had zoster do indeed have some scars, and this can be quite a problem if they appear on the face.

Treatment of the pain (called post-zoster neuralgia or PZN) is extremely difficult. Chronic pain relievers are the only proven help, but dermatologists and neurologists are now trying other substances, such as antidepressants, Dilantin (phenytoin, a drug used for seizures), Taractan (chlorprothixine, a tranquilizer associated with decreased pain), and Haldol (haloperidol, a drug used in psychiatric disorders). At least it would be worth a try asking your dermatologist how the trials of these drugs are progressing.

Newer therapy revolves around the use of the juice of the pepper plant in a cream called Zostrix and the stronger Zostrix-HP. It is rubbed on the aching area several times daily and will deplete a chemical (called substance P) that transmits pain. This over-the-counter medication is very effective in helping with the pain.

Patients with PZN are willing to go anywhere and try almost anything, but I'd caution you to try a medicine only after some testing has been carried out showing effectiveness. One of the most dreaded complications of shingles on the face is that they might affect the cornea, or clear part of the eye. They usually do this if the tip of the nose is affected and actually has had blisters on it. This means that the nasociliary branch nerve has been affected, and that's the important one that supplies the cornea. And if the shingles virus infects the cornea, you're in trouble. (Ophthalmologists use potent antiviral ointments for this.) Other than that, you shouldn't have to worry about corneal involvement, even if the lids are severely involved. But most of us will consult an ophthalmologist to check on the eye condition of patients with zoster around the lids, just to be safe.

Impetigo

Impetigo (often mistakenly called "infantigo") is an infection of the skin by dangerous strep or staph bacteria. These bacteria can cause sore throats as well. Many children eventually have an episode or two of impetigo during the early years when young immune systems are developing.

Summertime is the worst time for impetigo. The heat makes moist skin fertile ground for the support of pathogenic (disease-producing) strains of bacteria. And exposed skin of children with infections enhances the spread of bacteria; that's why impetigo is thought to be so contagious.

Impetigo is a blistering disease. The spots start as reddish flat or bumpy spots that rapidly progress to blisters. The blisters break easily, weeping a clear, yellowish, infectious fluid that dries, forming the classic "honey-colored" crusts that tip off the dermatologist to the diagnosis.

While the infection of impetigo is seen as a local problem, some strep bacteria that cause it can also cause an inflammation of the kidneys known as nephritis. This risk is minimized through the use of oral antibiotics, which must be taken for a full ten days for adequate protection.

Topical antibiotics also will help impetigo heal faster, but most dermatologists prescribe oral antibiotics to ensure that any pathogenic staph bacteria are completely wiped out and to prevent nephritis developing from the strep bacteria. If topical antibiotics are used, the newer Bactroban seems to be the most effective ointment for this. It is applied to the spots and surrounding areas two or three times daily. Here are some general tips, though, that might help to prevent impetigo. If your child seems susceptible, use an antibacterial soap for your family (though you should keep in mind that such soaps can be overly drying in winter) such as Safeguard, Shield, or Dial.

Encourage your children to avoid contact with any children who have skin sores of any type. Contact with such sores causes impetigo. Tell your kids about the dangers of skin-to-skin contact with anyone who has sores.

If anyone in your family has frequent sore throats or nasal sores, ask your doctor to check them for pathogenic staph or strep; a family carrier could be seeding the disease among the children.

Make sure that any crusted sores on your children are examined early by a doctor. Treating one child early can prevent impetigo from developing in the others. If your child does contract impetigo, be sure to seek treatment before the child infects others.

Jock Itch

There was a guy in medical school who shook the entire first row of seats while constantly scratching a groin itch. The annoyance caused by this probably gave me my first hint that I was interested in dermatology. Anyway, this fellow was dubbed "Itchy" by his classmates, until he got to his dermatology rotation. There his attending physician offered some help.

It turned out that the fellow had had "jock itch" for twelve years! Imagine his surprise when a month of special antifungal pills made his lifelong scourge vanish. But you know how nicknames stick. Some of his classmates still call him Itchy.

In this section, I'm going to teach you everything you ever wanted to know about some troublesome problems, like jock itch, related predominantly to males.

Jock itch is a catchall term for over three different types of groin rash. The major one is tinea cruris, or fungus of the groin. It's usually a red rash seen in teens and older patients, almost always men. Usually, a fairly distinct reddish border is seen with tinea cruris. The border may be slightly raised, or swollen, and tends to be somewhat uneven in its outline. It rarely, if ever, crosses the crural fold. That's the fold where the legs attach to the groin. In other words, it almost never strikes the scrotum. It's treated with the medicines we are discussing for the other fungi, such as ringworm and foot fungus. It's fairly easy to clear up, but it can come back quite easily if the feet are infected with a fungus. Have them checked, too, and treated if necessary.

However, moniliasis, a yeast infection quite common in men, does cross the crural fold onto the scrotum quite often. When there's a rash of moniliasis on the upper inner thighs, it's usually a spotty redness with what's known as satellite papules, or tiny, distinct bumps around the edges. These are usually separate from the main body of the groin rash. It's treated with anti-yeast medicines such as Lotrimin, Loprox, and Spectazole. Sometimes an older, but very effective, medicine, Fungizone, is used. All these medicines (except Lotrimin) are obtained only through prescription.

The third common infectious cause of jock itch is erythrasma. This is an infection caused by a bacterium called *Propionibacterium minutissimum*. The most peculiar fact about this organism is that it secretes a chemical that glows coral red in the presence of a black light called a Wood's light, and that's the way dermatologists make the diagnosis. It's commonly treated with topical and internal antibiotics, which kill off the infecting bacteria quite rapidly.

ℰKeratosis ℰPilaris

A "GIFT" FROM PARENTS

Many patients both young and old complain of little raised, natural skin-tone bumps on the upper outer arms and some on the fronts of the legs. They are often seen in family members, too. These small, spiny, skin-colored bumps around hairs on the backs of the arms are called keratosis pilaris. They are a harmless projection of dead skin cells from the hair follicle opening that can be quite a nuisance, having what we call autosomal dominance, that is, occurring in about 50 percent of the progeny of a patient with the disease.

However simple the condition seems to be, it's one of the most difficult to treat. Most useful has been the polyester nonmedicated sponge (the Buf-Puf) used with slightly acid sulfur soaps for removing the scale. After washing with the sponge and this special soap, you should dry thoroughly and lavishly apply a moisturizing lotion to soften the hard, scaly bumps. The best lotion for this is one called LacHydrin, a prescription moisturizer from the Westwood Company. Other good nonprescription lotions, which you may want to try first, are Lacticare and LacHydrin 5, the milder form of the prescription lotion.

Mild to moderate sun exposure can also help this condition resolve, but remember that sun exposure causes other damage to your skin, so I would approach sun therapy for keratosis pilaris very moderately, if at all.

Some patients have an even more extensive and slightly more severe form of keratosis pilaris called inflammatory keratosis pilaris. That means the bumps are accompanied by redness and itching. The treatment I mentioned above should help adequately, but sometimes even antibiotics are necessary to help suppress the inflammation and possible bacterial infection that can result in

129

these red, itchy bumps. In these cases, it's more like treating acne than routine keratosis pilaris.

Treatment for inflammatory KP (as it is called) is long and drawn out. It consists of using oral antibiotics, topical softening agents such as LacHydrin and Retin-A cream of various strengths, as well as occasional vitamin A used orally for a short term in moderate doses. Remember that oral vitamin A can be toxic in high doses for a long period of time, so be sure to contact your dermatologist and discuss this at length.

Laser Treatment for the Skin

NOT JUST FOR STAR TREK

Just the word "laser" makes us think of Star Trek medicine. However, laser surgery is much more accessible than that . . . and *you* could be a candidate. It is usually not as expensive as you would think. However, it can be painful in some cases, necessitating general anesthesia. Laser surgery is in a constant state of change, so don't take this as the last word on the subject. There are many different lasers suited to different tasks, with more and probably better lasers on the horizon.

The carbon dioxide (CO_2) laser was the first laser to be used extensively. The major functions of this laser are to cut and destroy ("ablate") tissue. When the CO_2 laser is used to cut, it basically functions as a scalpel blade—slicing through tissue. The only real advantage is less bleeding, as the edges of the wound are slightly cauterized during incision. When used to ablate tissue, the CO2 laser has been used to destroy numerous types of skin growths and neoplasms, most notably warts. This also works well but is not the only way to treat warts, and it requires a prolonged healing period. The carbon dioxide laser, like other surgical methods, can leave noticeable scars. Carbon dioxide lasers have been used to remove tattoos, but they leave scars and have been replaced by other lasers for this use. CO_2 laser usually requires local anesthesia of the area to be treated. There is now work indicating that "super-pulsed" CO_2 laser (the laser beam is "cut" into very short bursts of laser energy to prevent too much heat energy developing in one place on the skin) can be used along wrinkles to soften them, as opposed to cutting them out. Time will tell.

Another laser, called the Q-switched ruby laser, is used to treat pigmented lesions (freckles, some forms of birthmarks) and black or blue tattoos. The beauty of this laser is that it is tuned to a wavelength that is absorbed by the pigment in the skin, and less so by the blood and water in the skin, so that the laser energy is concentrated in the pigment, thereby sparing the surrounding skin. Also, the laser energy comes out in a short, powerful burst that is just enough to rupture the pigment without overheating the skin. There are several similar lasers (Q-switched alexandrite for tattoos, flashlamp-pumped 510 wavelength dye laser for freckles and age spots) that also work nicely. All of these lasers rarely cause scarring but can cause some discoloration of the area that can last for months (or even permanently). These laser treatments are the only way to treat tattoos without causing noticeable scarring, but can get expensive due to the multiple treatments needed (something not considered while getting a tattoo, I'm sure). Local anesthesia may be needed.

The last laser we'll deal with, one useful for a great number of people, is called the flashlamp-pumped 585 wavelength pulsed-dye laser (pulsed-dye laser). This laser is incredible for facial blood vessels (telangiectasias) and for port-wine stain birthmarks. The pulsed-dye laser is also a selective laser; it is on a wavelength that is preferentially absorbed by the color red. Therefore, the laser energy is absorbed by the red blood cells in blood vessels more than by the surrounding skin. This laser also gives off short powerful bursts of energy that are enough to "zap" the blood vessel without burning the surrounding tissue; scarring is virtually unheard of even after multiple treatments. Usually, a prescription anesthetic cream applied before laser surgery is all that is needed in adults. For lesions on children, or for large lesions, a local or general anesthetic may be needed.

Many adults get small capillary blood vessels (telangiectasias) on their faces, usually from accumulated sun damage. Some adults also get these from an inflammatory condition of the face called rosacea. For extensive facial vessels, one or two laser treatments can clear these nearly completely, without scarring. Although a tiny electric needle can be used also, it isn't practical for extensive vessels, and it tends to hurt more and can potentially cause tiny pinpoint scars. Laser works better for these telangiectasias.

For children or adults with port-wine stain birthmarks (those dark-red blotchy spots), multiple treatments are given every one to two months. Anywhere from two to more than ten treatments may be needed, depending on the darkness and thickness of the spot as well as the age of the patient.

The pulsed-dye laser is also being used for some warts that have resisted other treatments. We think the laser works by attacking the capillaries feeding the wart and by overheating the wart. This laser has also been used on psoriasis patches but is definitely *not* the first way to treat psoriasis.

Oh, did I mention that there is dark-purple, bruiselike discoloration of the treated areas for ten to fourteen days after pulsed-dye laser treatment. It's a bit hard to hide, too. But the results are worth it. Also, this laser hasn't been helpful for leg veins because leg veins are too deep under the skin and are too wide to be completely closed by the laser. Work is under way with other "machines" that may be useful for leg veins someday.

Don't be surprised if you need to go to a hospital outpatient surgery center for these treatments. Most of these lasers are too expensive for one office to buy. And don't be afraid to ask your dermatologist about your laser options—you could benefit from these new technologies, too.

$\mathcal{L}ice$

TEENS ARE A PRIME TARGET

Beware! All teenage skin problems are not acne! Teens suffer from a tremendous array of skin troubles that have nothing to do with acne even though the teens themselves sometimes think they do. To wit, Harry's story.

Harry, a nineteen year old, complained that he had "a constant battle with acne on strange parts of my body, including areas around my genitals."

"Acne in your groin?" I asked.

"Yep, I've noted little black dots on the skin of my groin and white dots actually on the hairs themselves. My family doctor gave me a prescription for it and told me it was an infection, but it has not gone away. Could it be something else?"

"Well, yes, I believe it could, Harry; indeed it could."

"Well, what then?" Harry asked.

"Lice. Pubic lice. Now, let's take a look and see what's 'bugging' you."

Harry dropped his trousers and revealed a massive infestation with pubic lice. They were crawling everywhere. The nits, or tiny eggs, were adherent to almost every one of his pubic hairs, and even as I watched, Harry could not stop scratching.

"What are they?" Harry asked impatiently.

"They're lice, Harry, no question about it," I said. "One of my residency mates had a very apt term for these itchy little critters. He called them 'crotch crickets.' "

I gave Harry a prescription for Kwell shampoo, which kills the lice, and told him to treat himself by sudsing up liberally every other day for a week. I also told him to send any sexual contacts he might have had to the health department to get checked for the same problem. Later, he told me that he was now very reluctant to call anyone a "louse" again. I've never figured out how his family doctor missed the diagnosis. Maybe he skipped his dermatology course in med school.

Teenagers have a fascinating plethora of changes occurring in their bodies that directly affect the day-to-day comfort of their existence. They're waging not only pitched battles to gain the recognition of their friends and schoolmates, but daily battles with an onslaught of new hormones. And these hormones can mark them for life.

Along with teenagers' new hormones come the whole complex series of emotional changes that lead to emotional involvement and sexual contacts, resulting in a host of "new" infectious diseases relating to direct or indirect contact. So, the skin of teenagers must return to war to fight these new invaders.

I am glad that often I get to see a teen early, so that when he or she gets an embarrassing problem later, I'm there, I hope as a trusted friend as well as a physician, to help them. I had treated one teenager, Mark, months previously for explosive cystic acne, and he now looked terrific. But this trip to the office was for something quite different. He appeared at our front office window and whispered to one of my staff, "May I please talk to Dr. Bark today; I don't have an appointment, and I think it's kind of important."

"Sure, Mark," said my receptionist, sensing a certain determined urgency in his voice, "I'll put you in Room 6 and ask Dr. Bark to drop in."

When I arrived, Mark was red-faced and frowning. "Dr. Bark," he said, not meeting my gaze, "I found this on my shoulder this morning and thought I'd bring it in to you. Can you identify it?" He held out a small, carefully folded notebook paper packet.

"I'll sure try, Mark," I said, wondering whether he might be suffering from delusions of parasitosis. That's a neurotic fear of things crawling on the skin, though Mark was far from neurotic. I carefully unfolded the tiny parcel to reveal a single hair with a single pubic louse, stiff alive and kicking, firmly attached to it.

Mark seemed destroyed when I told him he had "caught something from a 'friend.' " It took many minutes of explanation and a pledge not to inform his parents to calm him down. Finally, I managed to assure him that he'd survive this embarrassing problem, and so would his girlfriend. As it turned out, she was the first girl with whom he had had a serious relationship, so it was a very delicate problem.

In fact, when I think of how many skin problems can affect teens, it's really a wonder how any of us get to our twenties without getting some of them.

LICE—HOW TO GET THEM
AND HOW TO GET RID OF THEM

All of us want an "out" when we find out that we have a disease like lice. "Did I get it from a toilet seat?" we often ask. While theoretically you could have picked it up from a toilet seat, there would have to have been a fairly direct form of contact, that is, you would have had to sit down immediately after someone else with lice sat there. Lice do not like cold temperatures and rarely live long if they are deprived of body heat, so that the toilet seat theory is really difficult to believe with this problem and with venereal diseases as well.

A much more likely explanation is that you were sexually close to someone who had the infestation and some of the parasites crawled onto your skin.

Why do they call pubic lice "crabs"? Under a microscope they look like tiny crustaceans—shell, claws, and all.

Keep in mind that Kwell shampoo kills live lice and incubating eggs of lice (nits) almost immediately. However, you should be careful to wash your underwear in hot soapy water so that you don't get lice back from any nits that might have been deposited in the seams of your clothing. While this is usually a problem only with body lice, it can also be true for pubic lice.

The nits, while still firmly dry-cemented to the hair shaft, are dead as a doornail if you have used Kwell (lindane) in the prescribed manner.

Nits are very easily distinguished from flakes of dandruff by grabbing them with tweezers and trying to slide them up and down the hair shaft. If they do not slide, they are probably nits. If they slide very easily, they are most likely small flakes of dandruff.

Removing these small egg cases from the hairs is extremely difficult. The makers of Kwell (lindane) used to provide a small "nit comb" with their shampoo so that the nits could be combed out after treatment.

One dermatologist suggests a warm vinegar soak as a way to detach these tiny egg shells from the actual hair shaft. It is supposed to work very nicely. It certainly is cheap and should be harmless if you don't get it in your eyes (where it might sting).

School nurses are quite insistent on the cutaneous health of their children and will almost always refuse to admit children with remaining nits even though they have had the proper therapy prescribed by a dermatologist.

$\mathcal{L}iver\ \mathcal{S}pots$

OUT, OUT HAND SPOT!

One of the most troublesome conditions of aging is the appearance of many brown spots on the backs of the hands. These "birthday presents," as I like to call them, are usually flat, darkly pigmented brown spots on the backs of the hands. They're called "liver spots," because they were previously thought (incorrectly) to come from liver trouble.

Unfortunately, there are no lotions that will dependably remove them or make them lighter. The only way I know to do this effectively is through the use of cryosurgery. A light liquid nitrogen spray over the lesions will peel them off in one to three weeks, leaving a little red spot that will take a month or two to go away. The spots almost always turn back to normal skin color after a time, leaving you practically "spotless." Previously, liquid nitrogen wasn't widely available, but liquid oxygen was. So, since the cold of each is equally effective, dermatologists in this area used liquid oxygen for a long time. Shortly after I started practice, liquid nitrogen became the accepted standard.

A light spray is usually all that's needed to remove these spots. But remember, if any of your spots are red, scaly, or raised above the surrounding skin, you should definitely have them checked by a dermatologist. They could be many different types of spots.

Melasma

"I'm sorry, Doctor," said a patient, Jenny, "but a woman's skin is just not like a man's skin! My face is too dry to use regular acne lotions. I need a moisturizer. I need cosmetics. And for you to tell me that I cannot use them just will not work for me!" That statement, from an irate patient, expresses much of the bewilderment of women who encounter the advice and regulations of traditional dermatology. When, as a resident, I overheard her saying this in the office of a private dermatologist, I realized that not enough dermatologists think to give female skin the very special care it needs.

In this section, I will touch on many topics that have only traditionally been skimmed over by dermatologists, since we are mainly concerned with treating diseases rather than with the cosmetic needs of patients. But persons like Jenny, I found out, need special handling, diseased or not.

We know a lot about the peculiar mix of hormones and genes that surround and affect the skin of a woman. Many of the problems mentioned in this section affect women exclusively, but others also affect men. They are mentioned here because, in my experience, they are far more common in women. Take pigmentation, for example, an area where hormonal influences exert maximal effect.

THOSE ANNOYING TANNISH BLOTCHES

Thousands of women develop "pigmentation brown spots"—melasma—on their faces during their teens, twenties, and thirties. These annoying flat, tannish blotches can literally disfigure a woman, making normal social life virtually impossible. This so-called mask of pregnancy can make a woman look like a raccoon. Dermatologists think this altered pigmentation results from the hormone changes that accompany childbearing. Unfortunately, the mask of pregnancy is also a severe occasional side effect of taking birth control pills.

The actual brownish facial color of melasma results from deposition of excess color pigment, melanin, in the upper layer of skin, the epidermis. Unfortunately, most cases of melasma fade extremely slowly, if at all. Some women notice very slight fading with time, but I've seen the problem persist for years without any visible lightening.

For years women have turned toward over-the-counter creams to fade their facial pigment. These creams contain a minuscule amount of hydroquinone, a chemical that slows the output of melanin from the tiny skin pigment cells. However, the concentration of hydroquinone is so slight in these "medicines" that they take months to years to work, if indeed they ever do. In practice, they often don't. At least, I've never seen a case of melasma clear up with these over-the-counter fade creams.

A very effective remedy has been developed by the Neutrogena Corporation (the same company that makes Neutrogena soap for irritated or sensitive skin). The new agent is called Melanex. It's concentrated hydroquinone in a specially formulated lotion that penetrates to the exact level of the skin where the pigment is made. Supplied in a convenient pad-topped bottle, it's designed to be applied sparingly to the skin twice daily. To this date, it's the most effective depigmenting lotion I've ever seen. It's a prescription item, however, so you'll have to ask your dermatologist for it and for careful instructions on its use.

An important study in the *British Journal of Dermatology* in 1981 showed that doctors can often predict how well a patient would improve on hydroquinone therapy by testing her with a black light called a Wood's light. In most cases this light reveals whether you have the epidermal (surface) type of pigment or the dermal (deep) type. The former responds much better to Melanex than the latter does. Ask your doctor if he or she uses this test. It'll give you some indication of how well you can expect to improve. It seems that, in some people, the pigment cells are exquisitely sensitive to the effect of sex hormones. That means that even women who have not been pregnant may have enough of the required hormone around, possibly progesterone, to turn on their melanocytes.

Believe it or not, there are even some men who have melasma. And certainly they don't take the pill. But each of us has both male and female hormones. In those men with melasma, their tiny amounts of estrogen or progesterone must be just enough to turn on their facial-color cells, when combined with genetics and sun exposure. In the treatment of melasma, avoidance of sun exposure is not only important but crucial! I have never seen a patient's melasma improve without her taking great pains to keep the sun's rays off her face.

How do you avoid it? Sunscreens are essential. Melasma patients should use these lotions every day, because even the small amount of sunlight obtained going to and from the house and car can maintain the ugly pigment. In other sections of this book, you'll learn a lot more about protection from the sun in ways that really will save your skin.

Mohs Micrographic Surgery

After patients learn that they have skin cancer the next question is, "what can be done?" Although there are many treatments for skin cancers, the key to success for all of these therapies is to *completely* eradicate all of the cancer cells. If some of the cancer cells persist despite treatment, then the cancer regrows, much like a weed returns if its roots aren't pulled out. Mohs micrographic surgery provides the most precise and comprehensive method for tracing out and removing the roots of skin cancers resulting in the best cure rates of all available treatment options.

Having a precise method for tracing out the roots of skin cancers is important because they grow in unpredictable patterns and the cancer "roots" aren't distinguishable from normal tissue without the aid of a microscope. A skin cancer can be compared to an iceberg because only about one third of an iceberg sticks up above the surface and the submerged two thirds aren't readily visible. Because passing ships can't tell where the submerged part of an iceberg projects they steer well away to avoid a collision. In this analogy, if the captain of the ship had the advantages of a Mohs surgeon, it would be as if he had a team of scuba divers to mark the edges of the iceberg with buoys and the ship could then approach and go closely around the perimeter of the iceberg safely. In the case of Mohs micrographic surgery, by using the microscope to check all of the surgical margins, the surgeon can go closely around the tumor to remove it safely yet spare the maximum amount of unaffected surrounding tissues.

One important distinction of Mohs micrographic surgery is that the surgeon also acts as the pathologist. Frozen section microscope slides are prepared in the surgeon's office, and the surgeon reads the slides under the microscope. If cancer cells are present at the outside edges (surgical margins) of the removed tissue, the surgeon marks the location of the tumor on a tissue map. The tissue map tells the surgeon in which direction the cancer roots are projecting, and this guides the surgeon in removing small amounts of additional tissue. Efficiency, precision, and economy are optimized by the Mohs surgeon acting also as the pathologist.

Mohs micrographic surgery is very reliable and gives the highest cure rates of all cancer treatments. Cure rates for primary tumors (ones that haven't been treated previously) reaches 97–99% and even in cancers that have already failed treatment with other methods, Mohs micrographic surgery results in a 90–95% cure rate. Because of its reliability and precision it is used in difficult cases such as those that haven't been cured by other techniques or ones that have a pattern of invasive growth. It is used in areas where it is important to have both a high cure rate and the smallest defect possible such as the nose, ears, eyelids, lips, and face. A good example of this was the Mohs micrographic surgery performed on President Reagan to remove the skin cancer on his nose. Most cancers removed with the Mohs micrographic technique are either basal cell or squamous cell cancers because they are the most common. It is also used for less common skin cancers. Malignant melanomas are not routinely removed with the Mohs technique, but in special cases such as malignant melanomas on eyelids it is sometimes used to help preserve as much normal tissue as possible.

To explain the actual technique used in Mohs micrographic surgery we will describe the case of a fictitious patient, Mr. Tanswell. Mr. Tanswell had noticed a new bump on the side of his nose and mentioned it to his dermatologist, Dr. Bark. Dr. Bark listened to Mr. Tanswell and was immediately suspicious that he would find a skin cancer when he heard that the spot on Mr. Tanswell's nose bled from time to time and failed to completely heal. Dr. Bark noted a pea-sized bump on the tip of his nose and the bump had a grey shiny surface. Dr. Bark suspected that this was a basal cell carcinoma and recommended a biopsy. Mr. Tanswell asked some questions and particularly wanted to know why Dr. Bark wouldn't just treat the bump today if he thought it was a skin cancer rather than bothering with a biopsy. Dr. Bark explained that the biopsy would be a small sampling procedure which would leave a minimal, if any, scar. He explained further that if the papule turned out to be benign then he would be saving the patient from more extensive and more expensive surgery. On the other hand if it did turn out to be cancer, then the biopsy would give important information to plan the appropriate treatment. Mr. Tanswell agreed to the biopsy and Dr. Bark's nurse brought a few instruments into the exam room. Dr. Bark placed a few drops of Xylocaine (numbing medicine) just under the bump using a tiny needle and syringe. Mr. Tanswell felt a pinprick, but it faded within a few seconds as the medicine quickly numbed the spot. Using a scalpel, Dr. Bark painlessly shaved a thin sample of tissue from the bump and placed it into a specimen cup to be sent to the dermatopathologist. Mr. Tanswell inquired if Dr. Bark had started yet. He was pleasantly surprised that it was so quick, uneventful and painless except for the initial pinprick. A small spot bandaid was applied and Mr. Tanswell was released with the understanding that Dr. Bark's office would notify him of the results.

Several days later Dr. Bark reviewed pathology reports and noted that Mr. Tanswell's biopsy showed a basal cell carcinoma. Dr. Bark called Mr. Tanswell with the news and suggested that Mr. Tanswell have the cancer treated with the Mohs micrographic surgery technique. He explained that his colleague, Dr. Buker, performs this technique and that it is the best way to remove this cancer. An appointment was set and Dr. Bark asked Mr. Tanswell not to take aspirin or any aspirin-containing medicines for ten days prior to the surgery date. He explained that aspirin thins the blood and causes more bleeding during surgery and that it takes about ten days for the blood-thinning effects of aspirin to wear off. He told Mr. Tanswell that he may eat and drink normally before and after the surgery because it is performed under local anesthesia just like the biopsy procedure. He asked Mr. Tanswell to take his normal daily medicines on schedule as usual. He also asked Mr. Tanswell to wear comfortable, loose-fitting clothes and to bring a good book to read because there would be waiting periods of about one hour while the frozen section microscope slides are prepared and evaluated. He explained that if reconstructive surgery were required, Dr.

Buker performs most repairs on the same day as the cancer removal, but occasionally the repair may be referred to another specialist. He asked Mr. Tanswell to have a relative or friend accompany him on the day of surgery to handle the driving on the trip home.

On the day of surgery Mr. Tanswell and his wife came to Dr. Buker's office and Mr. Tanswell was shown to the minor operating room. A small amount of numbing medicine was injected around the skin cancer; then Dr. Buker surgically removed the affected skin. A dressing was placed over the wound and Mr. Tanswell was taken to join his wife in a private waiting area while the tissue was checked. Mr. Tanswell spent a total of 20 minutes in the surgery room and found the surgery itself to be painless except for the pinprick when the local anesthesia was administered.

In the lab the tissue was prepared by freezing it solid then cutting very thin microscope sections from all of the outside surfaces of the surgical specimen. Special stains were applied and Dr. Buker reviewed the slides under the microscope. In this case there were some cancer roots extending deep in the center of the wound and also some extending to the right edge of the wound. As he checked the slides Dr. Buker marked on the tissue map those areas where cancer roots extended deeper and wider. The process of preparing and checking the slides took about one hour.

Mr. Tanswell was returned to the minor OR and Dr. Buker explained that the cancer roots, which couldn't be seen with the naked eye, were extending deep and toward the right. Dr. Buker administered more local anesthesia. Then by using the tissue map to guide him, he took a small section of tissue from the deep and right margins of the wound but left the other areas that were "negative" alone. The surgery took fifteen minutes and again was painless except for the initial pinprick of local anesthesia. A dressing was placed and Mr. Tanswell rejoined his wife in the waiting area where they had some refreshments. After analysis of the tissue from this surgery (stage II), Dr. Buker found all margins to be negative and reported the good news to the Tanswells.

Mr. and Mrs. Tanswell were very pleased that the cancer was out, but they were concerned about scarring and what could be done to fix the defect on his nose. Dr. Buker explained that he recommended a skin graft for this situation, but he also reviewed several other options including natural healing without any repair which would leave a depressed scar, and a skin flap borrowed from higher up on Mr. Tanswell's nose which would cause some distortion to the nose. After their questions were answered, the Tanswells desired to have Dr. Buker perform the skin graft. Mr. Tanswell was again returned to the minor OR. Dr. Buker chose the crease behind Mr. Tanswell's right ear as the donor site for the skin graft and this area along with the nose defect were each prepared with surgical soap and local anesthesia. Dr. Buker first removed the donor skin graft and placed a few sutures to repair the donor site, then sutured the graft into place. A secure dressing was placed and the Tanswells were given post-op care instructions. The skin graft procedure took about one hour and, like the other surgeries, was painless except for the initial pinprick of local anesthesia. Mr. Tanswell planned to return in one week for suture removal.

The previous illustration points out that for each "stage" of Mohs micrographic surgery there is a brief surgery followed by about an hour wait for preparation and evaluation of the microscope slides. Although the average number of stages for most patients is only one or two, there are cases where five or more stages are required to completely trace out the tumor. For that reason patients are asked not to schedule other commitments on the day of their Mohs micrographic surgery in case their surgery requires many stages.

Moles and Shaving

What are the dangers in shaving over a mole or a birthmark on the face? If the mole sticks out a distance from the skin, the obvious hazard is cutting it recurrently. Does this cause cancer? Probably not, but it can cause confusion, in that any redness could be interpreted as a precancerous or frankly cancerous change by your physician. If that happens, then he or she is likely to recommend the complete removal of the mole. If it sticks up above the surface, therefore, I'd have my skin doctor see if it would be best to take it off via the shave biopsy technique, to lessen the effect of shaving over it. In any case, if a dark mole has been present since birth, most dermatologists would advise removal of it anyway.

Molluscum

Jane brought her four year old to me one day and said, "Looks like Troy has another selection from the 'Disease-of-the-Month' Club! Look at his rear."

I stood him on the exam table (after an appropriate amount of hand holding and reassurance), pulled down his tiny Bermudas, and found little Troy's bottom literally covered with tiny dots of an infectious virus called molluscum contagiosum. Viral, bacterial, and yeast infections are the most common childhood diseases. Why? Because just as a child learns the ways of adults as he or she grows, the diminutive immune system is learning what is self and what is nonself, what is foreign and what is familiar. But in order to learn to protect the child's young body, each substance, infecting agent, or antigen must be experienced at least once. And that's why so many children get warts, molluscum, impetigo, diaper rashes, and a host of other infections. Most of these infections do heal without a trace, but you must know that some, such as impetigo, can have serious consequences if left untreated. We'll talk more about such consequences elsewhere.

CAUSE AND BEST TREATMENT

Molluscum spots (like those on Jane's son, Troy) are caused by a large, brick-shaped virus that makes tiny one- to three-millimeter flesh-colored or pearly bumps grow on the skin. Molluscum means "soft body." That refers to the fact that these spots are not as hard and scaly as warts.

The second part of the name is "contagiosum," and you already have a sense for what that means. Anyone who touches this can grow his or her own set of molluscum lesions. They really like to grow in soft skin areas under armpits on children, but in adults they often occur in tender groin areas. Their propensity to strike the genital areas in adults has earned them the title of venereal disease, but that's really a misnomer, because most cases occur in children and are therefore unrelated to sexual contacts.

Many pediatricians question the need for treatment of molluscum contagiosum. They sometimes feel that, since they go away eventually, there's no need for vigorous therapy. But often the child whose spots go untreated will spread the disease to his or her friends, just by simple hand-to-hand contact. So we usually treat them when we find them.

Treatment is directed at removing a small kernel of virus from the center of the bump, called the molluscum body. Once this is gone, the spots resolve without scarring. The molluscum body exudes virus out of the center of the lesion like a small volcano, and that's what causes them to spread. Results of one experiment suggested that these bumps resolved just by pricking them with a needle, but I've never been able to reproduce that success.

In the old days, dermatologists advised patients to sharpen a fingernail and flick off the bump, but this often resulted in infection. A successful modification of this was developed, however, in which the bump is frozen lightly with a cold spray and then scraped off with a tiny curved knife blade called a curette. This works, but will occasionally cause scarring.

In my experience, the most efficient removal requires cryosurgery (freezing) with liquid nitrogen. The nice part is that these spots don't need to be frozen as firmly as warts and therefore don't hurt quite so much. It's not necessary to scrape the lesions; an extremely light freeze is all that's needed. They resolve beautifully with this treatment, without scarring.

Sometimes we use chemicals applied to the skin to cause some irritation, because it seems that sometimes the slightest irritation will result in the immune system's recognizing the virus as foreign, and it will then shed the lesions. Often, the children are brought into my office with some of the lesions already reddened and seemingly "infected," but this is the earliest sign that this particular bump is being healed by the body and will ultimately go away in a few days.

Often, for reasons we do not know, a reddish, scaly eczema accompanies the virus bumps. Could this be the body's earliest reaction to this virus? No one knows yet. Time may tell us lots more about the immunology of the human body through studying such innocent diseases as molluscum contagiosum.

Neurodermatitis and the Itchy Neck

HEALING IT FOR GOOD

Occasionally, eczema strikes the neck, especially the back of the neck. You've probably seen people scratching the backs of their necks from time to time. Often this is a condition that the early dermatologists called neurodermatitis.

Neurodermatitis is another one of those more or less psychodermatological terms. The real name for this disease is lichen simplex chronicus, a Latin term meaning "skin that thickens and scales due to long-term scratching." It usually starts out as a minor itching place on the back of the neck and scalp area. Scratching the spot damages the skin a little, and it heals ever so slightly thicker than before. That's because the skin is trying to protect itself by thickening. As healing progresses, the itch fibers in the skin are activated again by slight scar contraction in the damaged area. The new itching causes more scratching, damage, thickening, healing, and itching, and so on, and on, and on!

This is the itch-scratch cycle, and it can continue incessantly unless something happens to interrupt it. Usually, that something is a cortisone gel, cream, or liquid, which can finally halt the vicious itch-scratch cycle. Often we request that patients cut all the white free edges off their nails, so that there's essentially nothing there with which to scratch. We also ask patients to rub a little medicine into the area with the flat of their finger pad every time the spot itches. In this way, they do a modified "scratch" and apply their medicine at the same time.

149

Poison Ivy

LEAVE THESE LEAVES ALONE

"Leaves of three, leave it be!" Everyone's heard that old adage, but unfortunately, not enough of us heed its wise advice. There are few more uncomfortable patients than those with a severe case of poison ivy.

If you doubt how prevalent this affliction is, just look at the full shelf of over-the-counter remedies for it in the drugstore. It seems as if a new remedy springs up each year. Poison ivy is a problem, certainly, but one that can be prevented and treated very effectively if it does occur.

Poison ivy is a form of allergic contact dermatitis. This means that the skin gets allergic to the thick oily resin of the poison ivy plant. In order to do this, the resin from the broken leaf of the plant must streak across the skin. The resin can also be picked up by items such as tools, clothing, shoes, dogs, cats, golf clubs, and so forth, that have touched the resin and have not been cleaned thoroughly afterward.

FACTS AND FALLACIES

Scientists have found substances similar to poison ivy resin in Egyptian mummy tombs, and even after 3,000 years, the substance can still cause dermatitis! But it's really not hard to get rid of. Since the substance that causes the allergy is a thick oily resin, soapy water washes it away completely. No special soap is needed. Some people foolishly resort to using chlorine bleach, turpentine, and gasoline for removing poison ivy. This is completely unnecessary and can be quite irritating to the skin.

Realize that there is no way that the blister fluid from poison ivy skin lesions can cause disease in another person or, in fact, even spread it on the victim if the lesions have been washed with soap and water since initial contact with the resin.

Of course, this probably was not true in the old days when that folk tale got started. In those difficult days, people washed only about once a week. After several days, when their blisters began to weep, they still had the sticky resin that had not been washed off. So they indeed got new spots of poison ivy from the blister fluid, but this was purely by accident.

Remember: Be sure to wash off any item—animal, child, tool, or anything else—that has come in contact with the poison ivy resin, and you'll get fewer and fewer lesions instead of spreading the spots.

Since poison ivy is a disease of the immune system, it takes a finite length of time, usually two days or so, if a patient has had the disease before, to erupt on the skin in the classic streaked, red, itchy blisters. For this reason, dermatologists often call poison ivy the "Tuesday disease," because most cases show up in our offices on a Tuesday or Wednesday following picnics or outings on weekends.

There are even some dermatologists who refer to poison ivy as "the widow's weed." Widows often go out to their husbands' grave sites on Sunday afternoons to tend the grass and overgrowth around the graves. Here they often come in contact with poison ivy. Always be careful in clearing underbrush, since poison ivy often thrives in these areas.

Unnoticed exposure to poison ivy has been recognized by dermatologists for many years. Dr. Alexander Fisher, a renowned contact dermatitis specialist, is adept at tracking down contact exposure to weird substances, including various plants. He once had an elderly woman patient with an extremely tough case of apparent skin allergy. He suspected poison ivy but could not find the source. Finally, at lunchtime one day, Dr. Fisher went out to the patient's house and searched for sources of contact exposure. Every room in the house proved clean as a whistle. As he was leaving, the lady asked him if he would come see her beautiful growth of English ivy that she had cultivated for many years. As they rounded the corner of the house, Dr. Fisher gasped at what he saw. Her "English ivy" was a pure, undiluted culture of poison ivy plants. She had very carefully cultivated her "ivy" over the years, trimming, watering daily, and fertilizing it. After each exposure she developed more dermatitis. She apparently never realized it was due to her "English ivy" because of the delay between exposure and development of the rash.

There are people who are known to develop poison ivy dermatitis even after years of thinking they cannot get it. The immune system is pretty smart. It learns how to recognize a substance as a foreign, allergy-causing agent. That culmination of the training of the immune system can occur at any time, even after years of intermittent exposure.

BEST TREATMENTS

Avoidance is the best way to treat poison ivy. Admittedly, this is hard to do because of the varying look of the plants from time to time. Sometimes it grows as a shiny, three-leafed vine, and sometimes it stands alone like a tiny shrub.

Calamine is the age-old remedy for poison ivy. It does dry the lesions slightly and sometimes calms itching. But most of us feel that it really just covers up the sores so they're not so apparent. Personally, I think it's not worth the mess. As a matter of fact, no one has ever improved upon tap water soaks to help speed along healing of the blistering stage of poison ivy. Note that I said tap water. It doesn't help a bit to add anything to it (although some southern dermatologists recommend adding a small amount of bourbon to the tap water and then drinking it!). But clear water compresses without soap do help the acute stage.

Using topical hydrocortisone on poison ivy lesions functions more to mask the diagnostic signs of the disease than it does to help the itchy rash. In fact, the amount of hydrocortisone in the available over-the-counter cream is much too low to help the severe dermatitis of poison ivy. However, it can modify its appearance so that when you do see a dermatologist, an exact diagnosis may not be possible, since the skin rash can then look more like hives than like poison ivy. In some cases it is almost impossible to tell the difference except by watching the untreated lesions over a few days. When they blister, the correct diagnosis becomes obvious. There is one classical tip-off to poison ivy that we dermatologists use all the time to make the diagnosis instantly. If you have a rash that runs in straight streaks on your body, or is present in one part of the body that contacts another part of the body where you also find the rash, then think of poison ivy as the culprit. For example, the leaves often brush over one's arm, making streaks of the disease a couple of days later, or if it is initially seen on the thigh, the other thigh may have an identical spot of redness, blisters and itching. We dermatologists sometimes call this a "kissing lesion," because the contaminated skin of one area or body part touches that which is exactly adjacent to it. Look for these tip-offs and you may save yourself a doctor's visit.

You should also know that using topical antihistamines and numbing agents such as those ending in "-caine" or "-dryl" can result in worsening of your dermatitis if you get allergic to various substances in these medications. This includes vitamin E, which can cause severe dermatitis if an allergic reaction develops because of its use.

Amazingly, many patients get poison ivy from their firewood in the depths of winter. They think, mistakenly, that the logs are entangled by simple vines, but these vines are often poison ivy branches. Remember, the stems of the poison ivy plant still contain active resin even in the coldest of winters. That means if you carry in branches of poison ivy with your logs, you can look like a red blistered balloon a couple of days later.

Some patients have told me that most of the over-the-counter remedies work quite well within two weeks to heal attacks of poison ivy. This is a classic example of a mistaken "cause-and-effect" relationship. While many products available without a prescription may seem to help, these agents probably do nothing to improve upon the rate of healing of the poison ivy. If you would just let your case of poison ivy go untreated for a while, you would then see that the poison ivy rash decreases dramatically in almost *every* case within two to three weeks.

Pores (Enlarged)

DON'T PORE OVER YOUR PORES

Most enlarged pores on the facial skin are the result of one's unlucky ancestry more than anything else. And when you stop to think of how many thousands of women (and men) complain about their enlarged pores, it's truly a wonder why we don't often see large pores on others. What I'm trying to explain is that pores are rarely, if ever, visible to other people, but in this day and age of the great "magnifying mirror" society, most people can enlarge their images enough to spot the proverbial "nit on a gnat"!

If you insist on having something done to enlarged pores, first try Clinique's fabulous Pore Minimizer Makeup. It's great for hiding pores and making you look a lot smoother than you think you are.

Pregnancy

PUPPP—CURIOUS CONDITION OF PREGNANCY

The initials PUPPP stand for pruritic urticarial papules and plaques of pregnancy. This is an extremely itchy rash that starts like a very severe case of hives over the thighs and abdomen during late pregnancy. In fact, it can start in and around stretch marks. It often looks like hives, with large accompanying flat spots. PUPPP itches like crazy. And it's this itching which usually bothers mothers-to-be enough that they seek treatment.

This particular rash doesn't affect the baby's health (nor does it apparently cause the baby to itch), but it is an awful nuisance.

The treatment for PUPPP is topical cortisone, usually in cream or lotion form. Extreme cases can be settled down with antihistamines and even internal cortisone if the obstetrician and pediatrician agree it's okay. The rash goes away spontaneously at delivery or shortly thereafter, but a woman can get it again with her next child. We don't yet know the exact cause of PUPPP. Some factor produced by the baby or the placenta has been theorized as a cause, but never proved.

STRETCH MARKS AND PREGNANCY

The tremendous elasticity of the skin has been a constant wonder for thousands of years. Imagine the incredible stretching force of the pregnant abdomen; it's a miracle that the baby doesn't stretch right through. The skin performs admirably in shrinking down after delivery, usually taking only a few days to get back most of its normal tone, but almost all women are left with some permanent stretching that will not go away.

Stretch marks, or striae, are actual scars in the dermis, or second layer of the skin, in response to the stretching forces of preg-

155

nancy. When the collagen, the strong supporting network of the dermis, is pulled almost to the breaking point, the skin very wisely starts to lay down new layers of collagen fibers to add strength. This results in the classic stretch mark we all know and hate.

Of course, everyone knows about the stretch marks related to pregnancy, but many patients ask about the stretch marks most people get during the normal pubertal weight gain. These are usually around the hips and thighs, but can sometimes encircle the entire leg.

Another type of stretch mark is the type acquired by weightlifters. These "starburst" striae radiate outward from the armpits, and progressively worsen as the weightlifter builds muscle mass in the shoulder areas.

One last type of stria deserves mentioning. If you develop reddish-purple stretch marks that don't ever fade back to the usual ivory-white coloration, you should show them to your doctor. They could be a sign of a serious hormonal imbalance called Cushing's syndrome. Be sure you show this type of stretch mark to a physician.

Stretch marks commonly undergo some inflammation during their lifetimes. Usually, this is only a mild redness, but sometimes it's bad enough to cause quite a bit of itching. This is about equivalent to our grandparents saying that "if it's itching, it's healing," in that your body's trying to "heal" a dangerously stretched place in the skin. During this process, the contraction of the scarred stretch marks stimulates the itch fibers in the skin.

More important, the itching in stretch marks is often the result of an allergy to something being applied to the skin surface. This could be anything from an allergy to lanolin to a reaction to vitamin E, a frequent skin sensitizer.

There's been reported a curious "dermatosis of pregnancy," a rash acquired during pregnancy that involves striae. It's got the strange name of PUPPP, and it is discussed elsewhere.

There's no magic cream or lotion you can apply to the skin that will correct stretch marks. If there were such ingredients, there'd be no striae!

How do you get rid of stretch marks then? You don't. But they often become less obtrusive with time, and plastic surgeons can do wonders in hiding them. If yours really are noticeable, then you should consult a plastic surgeon.

$\mathcal{P}$soriasis

BEATING PSORIASIS—
HOW TO LIVE WITHOUT LEAVING
A TRAIL OF SCALES

"Joe," said our department chairman on my first day on the dermatology rotation, "today you'll learn the cardinal sign of psoriasis. Somewhere in this clinic, there's a severe psoriatic. I want you to find him."

"Sure," I said naively, "no problem. Just let me look through these charts in the wall rack, and I'll find him in a minute."

"Whoa!" he exclaimed. "No charts; just stand right here and find him."

"Hmmm," I mumbled, with sweat now forming on my palms. "I'm afraid I haven't had my X-ray vision tuned up lately."

"Look around, Doctor, the clues are here!"

I glanced down the long hallway leading to our exam rooms. All the doors were closed, and except for the unswept carpet, nothing was . . . unswept carpet? Unswept carpet! That was it! Leading all the way down the hall was a long trail of branlike scales tracking right into Room 12.

"Room 12?" I asked, with somewhat less than impressive confidence. "Absolutely," the chief asserted. "That patient drops enough scale each day to enable you to track him anywhere! Now go see him firsthand. It's Mr. Williams, one of our chronic psoriatics."

Although not every psoriatic is as scaly as poor Mr. Williams, tremendous scaling can occur if psoriasis gets out of hand. The chairman's "find the psoriatic" lesson taught me about the torment of this dreadful disease. Let's consider some of the many questions on the minds of psoriatics.

SCALES ON YOUR PERFECT SUIT

The "heartbreak of psoriasis" strikes 1 to 5 percent of all of us. Virtually everyone has seen someone with it. In ancient times psoriasis was often confused with leprosy so that psoriasis victims tended to live the lives of outcasts. The rare tendency for psoriasis to undergo spontaneous remission may even account for some of the "miracle cures" in early religious history.

Scaling and redness are the hallmark of the disease. A quick look at the exact skin defect in psoriasis explains why. In normal skin the epidermis remakes itself from top to bottom about every thirty days. Ordinarily, the dead skin is constantly being sloughed off in an orderly fashion from the uppermost layer, the stratum corneum.

Imagine a perfectly fitting suit, renewing itself constantly and never wearing out. Skincredible! But in psoriasis lesions, called plaques, the skin speeds up its own replacement, so that its entire thickness is reproduced every three days. Ten times as fast as normal skin. No wonder it scales!

The scaling of psoriasis is usually worst on the knees, elbows, genitalia, scalp, and between the buttocks. It is often a thick, whitish scale that early dermatologists called an "asbestos" or "silvery" scale because of its flaky, whitish-gray texture.

Often, the fingernails have small indentations or dot-sized dimples in the nail plates called pits. While occasional pits are normal, an increased number of pits, even ridges, due to lines of pits across the nail, may mean you've got the disease.

Occasionally the scaling spreads from localized areas to the usually normal areas of the skin. Sometimes it covers the entire body, resulting in a condition called exfoliative dermatitis, which means "shedding of the skin." It can be a life-threatening problem, even involving heart failure. This happens when the severe inflammation of psoriasis causes the superficial skin blood vessels to open up wide. This massive dilatation of the miles and miles of skin blood vessels causes the effective blood volume of the body to decrease. Then the heart pumps even harder to try to supply the internal organs with blood and eventually wears itself out. This is one of the few times that psoriasis can be fatal.

Patients with exfoliative dermatitis feel cold, too, because all the wide-open blood vessels conduct the vital heat of the body to the surface. That's why these patients often shiver, even in the heat of summer. Remember, red skin in a psoriatic can indicate the presence of exfoliative dermatitis, a true dermatologic emergency. If this happens, see your doctor immediately!

CONTAGIOUS—NEVER!

Along with the original "leprosy" fallacy about psoriasis, there are many other fallacies that should be dispelled. Psoriasis is not contagious. It's not an infection. Psoriatics are not unclean. As a matter of fact, one chief of dermatology at a large medical center illustrates this quite graphically to his new residents. He makes a bold point of his immediate warm handshake with even the scaliest of psoriatic patients, signaling with a quick commanding glance that the physicians-in-training should jump to follow his lead.

In fact, you can catch virtually nothing from an inflicted psoriatic. So if you know a psoriatic, or if you have the disease, stop worrying about catching it or spreading it to others. It may make a miserable disease a little more tolerable for the victim.

GENES WILL TELL

Psoriasis is not an allergy, nor is it a problem primarily caused by "nerves" or emotions, although stress does seem to play a sizable role, as I'll mention when I talk about treatment.

Unfortunately, there is one way in which the disease can be passed on—through inheritance. Almost 80 percent of my psoriatic patients have an affected relative. But there's no way to predict whether you will pass on the disease to your offspring. On the other hand, some psoriatics are known to have no relatives with the disease.

Long ago I learned firsthand about the hereditary nature of psoriasis when a biologist friend named Rob brought in his six-year-old daughter. She had reddish scaly spots on her chest and some minor scaling on her elbows. Although I considered psoriasis in the diagnostic list, the December weather led me to dub her problem xerotic eczema (dry irritated skin patches) commonly seen in winter.

But when they returned three weeks later with new spots, her knees also had small patches with thick, whitish scale. A thorough check of her fingernails revealed numerous tiny pits, confirming psoriasis. Thorough questioning about relatives revealed no trace of the disease.

You can imagine my dismay almost a year later, when Rob brought in his second child, a tiny towhead named Darren, with scaly ears and scalp. I ever so cautiously dubbed this seborrheic dermatitis, an inflamed itchy dandruff condition, but I was really hoping against hope that it, too, wasn't psoriasis. I raised the possibility with Rob that Darren had psoriasis, but I hesitated to alarm him unduly unless the signs and symptoms worsened. Unfortunately, Darren's ears developed the thick, reddish scaly plaques that heralded the onset of the disease.

Not until two years later did I discover how important inheritance was to Rob's kids. Our office air-conditioning was under repair on the hot summer day when he brought the kids in for a follow-up visit. Rob was in his shirt sleeves when I entered the room, and as I often do I shook his hand and gave him my usual friendly grip on the right arm and elbow with my left hand. As my fingers touched a scaly spot near his elbow, my friendly greeting turned to concern. I rotated his arm, stared at his psoriasis patch, and moaned a disappointed, "Not you too!" At last we knew the inheritance pathway of his kids' disease. Rob said he had had small "rough patches" on and off for years, but never related it to the kids' psoriasis.

NUTRITION AND PSORIASIS

A bewildering amount of psoriasis research has been done on its relationship to nutrition. In fact, basic research adds a new and innovative treatment approach every few years. Unfortunately, nutritional therapy and vitamin supplements are not among the ones that work. Long ago, proponents of the "turkey diet" for psoriasis found that the only thing it cured was the anemic wallets of the turkey producers. And I am sure that most of the psoriatics who tried it thought that it was indeed a "fowl" diet! But their psoriasis remained unchanged. Diet therapy is worthless as a cure for psoriasis.

There are no magic vitamin cures for psoriasis. In fact, there is one vitamin that can actually be harmful if applied topically—vitamin E. Topically applied vitamin E can cause a violent allergic sensitivity in the skin. This was discovered years ago when vitamin E was introduced in every form imaginable, from oils to deodorants to soaps. That's when our offices filled with victims of contact allergy to vitamin E.

There is, however, one topically applied vitamin preparation, called Dovonex (this is new) that can help. It is now FDA approved for use in psoriasis and works to cut down the scale and redness in many cases. It is safe, in that it is not a cortisone treatment, so the side effects of cortisones, such as skin thinning, will not occur. But it takes several weeks to months to see its effect, so be patient. And be patient with the expense, too—it's up there!

TREATING THE "HEARTBREAK"

The most widely accepted treatment is the use of potent topical cortisone creams and ointments applied frequently to the skin lesions. They work by decreasing blood flow to the psoriasis spots, a process called vasoconstriction. This process also decreases redness, skin turnover rate, and therefore the thick scales of the disease.

Certain regions of the body are very hard to treat. The lower legs are a tough nut to crack in psoriasis. The lesions here are more stubborn than anywhere else on the body. And soaps don't help. They usually dry, sometimes clean, and sometimes disinfect, but rarely do they help any skin disease get better. Their drying effect can greatly aggravate psoriasis, especially that on the extremities.

In general, if a patient with psoriasis has a tendency toward dryness on the arms and legs, I demand that he or she use nothing but gentle, superfatted soaps because of their mildness and moisturizing aspects. I also advise the patient to bathe (or shower) no more than twice a week, maximum. In between, spot-bathing can be done. Lotions help, especially if they have cortisone in them, but usually they must be compounded by your dermatologist to get them strong enough to help. Your dermatologist can see your spots, determine what they need, and mix a lotion tailor-made for your psoriasis, if necessary. But the moisturizing effect of over-the-counter lotions such as Complex 15 is obvious. They soften the lesions nicely if used frequently enough. If your dryness is tremendously excessive, you might ask your doctor for a prescription for a lotion called LacHydrin. This lotion sometimes causes a little stinging, but it is quite helpful in removing scale and moisturizing the legs and other tough areas.

HEADS—TOUGHEST TO TREAT

Severe scalp psoriasis is one of the most challenging diseases the skin can develop. It's tough! One of my patients came in with "scale so thick on my scalp that I sometimes can't see the hairs within it." I thought this patient was kidding until I peered through his hair onto a scalp covered with about a half inch of thick, whitish, sheet-like scale that covered his scalp nearly from one side to the other.

"What have you been doing to your scalp?" I asked.

"Well, it itches, Doc," he said, "and when it itches, I scratch it!"

"What do you use to do your scratching," I asked, " a garden rake?"

"You're close, Doc. Actually, and don't laugh when I tell you this," Jim said, "but I use our poodle's metal hairbrush to remove the scales!"

I fell back against the wall grabbing my chest and gasped. "A metal hairbrush! Look Jim," I explained, "nothing could be worse than scratching off those scales with a sharp, stiff metal brush." I told Jim that any irritation of psoriatic skin causes new plaques of psoriasis. This "Koebner reaction" often happens in minor scratches and wounds and on knees and elbows where friction is greatest (and, in fact, where psoriasis is greatest).

Almost every dermatologist has seen patients like Jim who have been scratching with hat pins, brushes, fingernails, nail files, pencils, and anything else they can get their hands on, not realizing that they're pouring gasoline on the fire of their disease.

I realize full well that itching is a very disagreeable sensation that demands that one scratch. But there's a way to do this that is less harmful and actually applies the medicine at the same time. Put a cortisone lotion or any of the cortisone medications your doctor may have given you on your flat finger pad and rub it into the spot that itches, rather than using a fingernail or other sharp object. This does not damage the skin, and you'll actually treat it repeatedly throughout the day any time it itches. In fact, the itching can be said to be your tiny alarm clock reminding you when to treat your psoriasis. Be sure to ask your doctor if this would be appropriate for use with your medications.

Most cortisone medications do not discolor the hair. Occasionally your doctor might choose to use thin cortisone lotions occluded with a plastic shower cap at nighttime to increase their potency. Studies show that this can make your medicine 50 to 100 times more potent, but do not do it unless your doctor specifically instructs you to do so.

Another agent you might try is Baker's P&S lotion. Used every night or every other night, this lotion will very effectively remove scales without your having to pull or scratch them off. Rub about thirty drops into the scalp at nighttime. Baker's P&S is a little tough to wash out in the morning, but it is a very, very effective scale remover.

Most patients have heard about the effective use of tar and tar shampoos on scalp psoriasis. Tar shampoos such as Pentrax, Ionil T Plus (two I like best), and many others are very effective treatments for those with brown or black hair, but for anyone with gray, white, or blond hair, they can cause quite a bit of golden-orange tinting. So if you want to try a tar shampoo, and you have white or gray or blond hair, then you should approach this carefully.

Psoriasis shampoos are meant to be scalp treatments. So they should be lathered once, rinsed off, lathered again, and left on for five to seven minutes while the medicine in the shampoo has a chance to work. After you have used psoriasis shampoos, you may use a rinse or conditioner of your choice on your scalp because the treatment from the shampoo has already been accomplished. Keep in mind, too, that a good smoothing rinse is wise to use because it will make it easier to comb your hair. The rinse removes the hair-to-hair friction, and this results in less trauma to the scalp, which could induce more psoriasis. The two most effective rinses are Ionil Rinse and Small Miracle by Clairol.

EAR PSORIASIS

Unfortunately, psoriasis loves ears. But over the years I've found a treatment that is nearly always able to clear ear canal psoriasis:

Halog solution. It's applied with a Q-tip to the ear canal as if you were actually painting the walls of the canal itself. The drops are put on the Q-tip (two or three drops will do), never dropped right into the ear. Many of us use this technique, so take this book to a dermatologist and ask whether you can try it. If it works, you've got it made! If not, you've put yourself in touch with a source of help who can advise you on what else you can use. During the acute stages of ear canal psoriasis, the Halog treatment is usually needed twice a day, with the frequency tapering off as you improve. However, take care to heed the old adage, "never put anything in your ear smaller than a football!" Never use a wooden-shafted cotton swab, and never put anything far into your ear. To do so is to invite disaster if you slip and damage your eardrum. Be advised that there are also other cortisone solutions that may be used like Halog, such as Lidex solution, Diprolene lotion, and others.

THE PUVA PROMISE—
SOME GOOD NEWS, SOME BAD

Psoriasis of the palms and soles, or palmoplantar psoriasis, is one of the most difficult and painful types of psoriasis. For some reason, a small percentage of patients get these small pus pockets and scale predominantly on the palms and soles rather than getting the usual body skin-type lesions.

While antibiotics sometimes help, it's often necessary to use cortisone topically for long periods and even internally on a periodic basis to keep this settled down. Of course, we would all like to get away from internal cortisone as much as possible because of its side effects, and a development in psoriasis therapy now allows us to do that.

The treatment is called PUVA. PUVA stands for Psoralen plus ultraviolet-A light therapy. This technique is called photochemotherapy because the chemical (Psoralen) makes the skin much more photosensitive. The medicine is given two hours before the patient undergoes controlled light exposure in order to give it time to lodge in the skin.

In photochemotherapy, the active drug binds to the DNA of the epidermis. You'll remember that the epidermis is the exact area where psoriasis occurs. This drug attracts ultraviolet light and stops the rapid multiplication of these cells that cause the thick scale and redness of the disease. Special precautions, tests, and light-tight glasses must be used with this treatment, and it's necessary to get two to three treatments a week at the onset. Ask your doctor about this therapy and its possible complications.

Does pregnancy help psoriasis, or make it worse? Sometimes pregnancy does help psoriasis. However, the course of psoriasis during pregnancy is so variable that an accurate prediction cannot be made.

More important, however, is the fact that the psoralens for the PUVA treatments is listed in the package insert as "Pregnancy Category C." Animal reproduction studies have not been conducted with psoralens. It is also not known whether psoralens can cause fetal harm when administered to a pregnant woman or if psoralens can affect reproduction capacity. In view of this "warning," I don't put any pregnant psoriatics on the drug.

To avert some of the difficulties with this treatment, some dermatologists are now using psoralens topically. This avoids the various complications of dosing the total body surface with the potent light, when only a fraction of the skin may be involved. There's no sense in exposing the skin to unnecessary damage in areas that do not have psoriasis. It also averts the need to wear protective glasses after the treatments. With systemic photochemotherapy, the glasses must be worn during sun exposure for twenty-four hours after UVA treatments. This is because the Psoralen binds to the protein in the lens of the eye and may cause damage (cataracts) if light of the UVA wavelength strikes it. PUVA treatment has been approved by the FDA for use in severe psoriatics.

THE COSTS OF TREATMENT

Unfortunately, the cost of modern-day medicine is not inexpensive, especially with regard to the cortisone compounds and other strange medicines we use so often in dermatology. However, an intensive psoriasis treatment program does provide the patient the ability to keep working and lead a productive life. In that sense, it can be said to be well worth the expense.

I have suggested on occasion that psoriasis patients go to university clinics or try to obtain public aid for psoriasis, but I have more or less stopped doing this. You see, most public assistance programs will supply only the weakest of medications to patients with skin diseases. Occasionally, however, in cases of severe need, exceptions to the rules are made, especially if your doctor will go to the trouble to request special help for you from your state agencies. If you have psoriasis and you need help with the cost of the medicines and treatments, ask your doctor; it's certainly worth a try.

So we come full circle right back to the private dermatologist who handles the brunt of psoriasis treatment in this country. Most doctors are reasonable people, and it is often possible to budget payments for dermatologic care and for medications; discuss it with your dermatologist. It is possible that he or she may modify your treatment, follow-up regimen, and medications in order to alleviate your costs somewhat.

There are also some very inexpensive medications that, although potentially hazardous in some ways, do have the benefit of being less expensive. Methotrexate is one of these (see the following section).

METHOTREXATE—TWO-EDGED SWORD

Years ago methotrexate (MTX), a medicine ordinarily used to treat cancer patients, was found to help psoriasis significantly in nearly every patient who took it when given by injection or by mouth.

However, after a while it was noted that some patients on MTX were starting to show changes in their liver, the organ that helps break down drugs and waste products in the body. Those patients who did incur liver damage were usually getting the MTX on a daily basis, whereas those who got the tablets on a once-a-week schedule incurred fewer problems. Now most patients are taking the pills once a week. Liver damage can still occur, and so can other reactions, such as depression of the blood cell count, so that a close follow-up is mandatory. Usually, the dermatologist will want to have a gastroenterologist or a liver specialist perform a liver biopsy before starting methotrexate. This allows your dermatologist to document whether you have a normal liver prior to the onset of MTX therapy. Periodic, sometimes weekly, lab exams are performed by dermatologists in order to follow closely any changes in liver or blood function. And no alcohol should be ingested during therapy.

But the medicine does work. And if you're interested in finding out more about MTX therapy for psoriasis, talk to your dermatologist, who should discuss thoroughly all the possible advantages and disadvantages (complications) of the medicine. It's not an easy drug to use, and patients taking it have to be carefully monitored. I urge you to cooperate with your doctor's recommendations in this regard.

PSORIATIC PENILE PLAQUES

Some men have quite severe psoriasis spots on the head of the penis. These spots get much worse after intercourse and take a long time to heal. Sometimes the tiny scales pull off and bleed profusely. Intercourse is a type of irritation that can induce a Koebner reaction right on the head of the penis (glans). The friction causes minor irritation, which is followed, over the next few days, by new and/or thicker psoriasis plaques.

Doctors often will put patients on medications, possibly a special, gentle medication for this soft skin area, which can help alleviate the condition. Adequate lubrication in the vaginal canal is also essential to keeping psoriasis-inducing friction to a minimum. Use plenty of K-Y Jelly, a water-washable lubricant, as a friction preventer. Some dermatologists also suggest that a cortisone compound be applied to the head of the penis prior to intercourse so that the lesions may be partially blocked from forming. However, the treatment for genital psoriasis is not perfect, and occasional bouts of abstinence may be necessary to allow healing.

NERVES, CANCER, AND PSORIASIS

A frequently asked question is whether psoriasis is a type of cancer. Is it cancer of the blood? Do nerves causes psoriasis? The fact is, psoriasis has nothing to do with cancer or blood diseases, except that a few of the treatments are somewhat the same for both diseases. But I think there really is something to the fact that some psoriasis patients get better if they are taken out of their stressful day-to-day environment. This was vividly demonstrated to me by a professor of dermatology at the Medical College of Georgia who suggested, "Joe, I'd like you to put Mr. Orvine in the hospital for a few days and do nothing for him but feed him and give him a place to excrete."

"Don," I said, "you've been working far too hard teaching us residents everything we need to know. I really think you must have lost your mind! Would you like me to run over and grab a shrink for you to talk to?"

"Joe, your trouble is that you've got no faith," Don replied. "Trust me for a change, Joe, and see what happens."

"But, Don," I exclaimed, "he'll get psoriasis everywhere if we just put him in bed and not treat him!"

"Trust me," Don said, "just trust me."

"You're the boss," I said, thinking how strange it was that such a superb clinician should go crazy so suddenly.

So we admitted the seventy-year-old man with generalized red psoriasis and tremendous scale everywhere, put him to bed, fed him, and did not apply one stitch of medicine other than to give him anti-itch medicines by mouth.

Amazingly, over the next few days our elderly patient's scaling decreased, as did his redness, and clear spots of normal-looking skin began peeping through the large areas of psoriasis.

"Don," I admitted, "I'm frankly amazed!"

"I'm not a believer in stress reduction helping much in dermatology," Don said, "but in psoriasis, it really has a terrific effect."

"Touché!" I exclaimed.

Since then, I've found it to be a constant truth that patients do better when their stress is reduced. This can mean trying to rearrange work so that it's less disagreeable and less stressful, or it can involve other stress-reduction techniques, but severe psoriatics should surely try it.

RELIEF FROM ITCHING

What can be done for the toughest spots? You've heard me talk about the Koebner reaction, in which more psoriasis is caused by scratching. To prevent this, the important thing is to get rid of the itching. Usually, when the psoriasis starts to improve, the itching does too. This means that patients must apply faithfully any medication the dermatologist has given them. Then as the psoriasis gets better, so will the intense itching.

As a help for the itching in the meantime, I suggest antihistamines such as Atarax, Claritin, and Tavist, which can calm the itching significantly while the patient waits for the spots to heal.

Of course, other treatments besides cortisone can be of help to psoriasis. These include the tar-type medications with or without ultraviolet light. Usually tar is applied overnight and an ultraviolet treatment is given the next day, but, more recently, modifications of the old tar derivatives have appeared for dermatologists' use.

One of these tar derivatives is a medicine called Drithocreme, an imported anthralin medication from England. Anthralin, while staining and sometimes irritating, can speed the healing of psoriasis tremendously. One type of anthralin (Dritho-Scalp), can be rubbed into the scalp at nighttime to improve the scalp disease. It's messy and can definitely discolor hair, so get exact instructions from your dermatologist before you begin to use this prescription medicine.

INFANTILE PSORIASIS

Frequently I hear that very young infants have contracted psoriasis. I've seen my youngest case of psoriasis at six weeks. The age of onset seems not to be at all predictable. But it surely is a lot tougher to treat in babies, because their tender skins won't tolerate some of the more potent medicines that work so well in adults.

PSORIASIS IN HISTORY

Until a few years ago, low-dose arsenic had been used successfully in treating difficult psoriasis. But since arsenic causes internal cancers and other problems many years after its administration, its practical use was restricted to the elderly, who would not be expected to encounter these late-appearing sequelae during their lifetimes. This just demonstrates how psoriasis therapy differs depending on the age groups under consideration.

PREJUDICE AGAINST PSORIASIS VICTIMS

The general public understands so little about the disease that prejudice and preconceived notions run rampant, making the psoriatic's life miserable. If I've dulled those prejudices even a little, I'll consider this book a success.

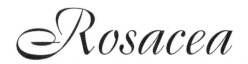

Rosacea

Rosacea is an inflammatory condition of the facial oil glands and the skin in between them. It is more common in middle-aged women than in men, although the prime example of rosacea in everyone's mind is the condition that caused W. C. Fields' bulbous nose and what he called "gin blossoms." These lesions were the cardinal signs of this condition, the telangiectasias or dilated blood vessels that are common in the disease.

For many years no one knew what influences initiated an attack of rosacea. It was known that a genetic tendency was present, but treatment was lacking. Sulfur lotions were the mainstay for this and for acne in teenagers. Thus rosacea became known for many years as "acne rosacea," although acne is different—in acne there is no inflammation between the follicles, and many acne patients do not exhibit the tendency toward easy flushing and blushing that rosacea patients have.

In recent years, a type of mite called *Demodex* has been implicated in causing rosacea, and a new preparation is available to kill off these facial parasites. Using this amazing gel, called Metrogel, along with the anti-acne antibiotic tetracycline, can allow the face to heal rapidly.

It is especially important to treat rosacea early to prevent chronic inflammation of the facial oil glands and enlargement of them, which causes a gradual enlargement of the tip of the nose (so-called drinker's nose).

Telangiectasias that remain after the disease is gotten under control may be treated with electrodesiccation (buzzing with an electric needle).

Foods have long been the subject of speculation as causes of rosacea. The most important food aggravants are hot liquids, which dilate the blood vessels of the neck and face, causing more flushing. Also, caffeine, sun, wind, heat, and cold all are bad for rosacea. Alcohol worsens the disease, thus the saying that this is a drinker's problem first and foremost.

Scabies

Scabies (rhymes with "rabies") is a contagious disease often called "the itch." It is an ancient disease. Scabies is an infestation by mites too tiny to be seen with the naked eye. These tiny creatures crawl around just beneath the skin surface, excreting material that causes stupendous itching, especially at nighttime. Scabies is passed from person to person by direct contact.

NAPOLEON'S DOWNFALL

The itch has a famous place in history. It probably lost the Battle of Waterloo for Napoleon. His whole army had the disease and was unable to rest adequately the night before the great battle. As a matter of fact, Napoleon himself had the itchy nuisance for years. Just think of all the paintings of Napoleon you have seen with his hand in his shirt. Historians say he was scratching the itch!

Scabies itching, usually worse at night, is most severe between the finger webs and under the armpits and in body folds, the navel area, and very frequently on the head of the penis, a soft spot that mites seem to love.

Scabies can't be definitively diagnosed unless we actually find evidence of the mites' presence. To do this, we scrape off one of the tiny suspicious bumps and apply a small drop or two of potassium hydroxide (KOH). The KOH causes clearing of the skin cells, allowing the protein case of the mite shell to be seen quite clearly under the microscope. Eggs and droppings from the mites can also be seen with great regularity during this test.

The incredible itching of scabies at night may result from the calming of daytime distractions, allowing the itching to surface into consciousness. However, some investigators feel that the mites actually move more at nighttime than they do during the day.

We may not know an answer for why patients itch when they have scabies, but itch they do. In fact, even after successful treatment of scabies, the itching can last for three or more weeks. We call this the "itch of infection." It is probably due to the dead bodies of mites and the products they leave embedded in the skin, until the skin has a chance to reproduce itself and shed the infected areas.

BEST TREATMENT

Treatment for scabies is relatively simple, but it has to be done exactly right. Usually this consists of the application of lindane lotion to all body skin of every infected family member for twenty-four hours, once a week, for two to three weeks. While these are general recommendations, almost every dermatologist has slight variations in the treatment for his or her own patients. For instance, some dermatologists do not treat infants with lindane. I don't, because a study some time ago showed toxic effects in animals who were bathed excessively in the lindane products. In such cases, Eurax cream and lotion or, better yet, Elimite cream can be substituted for lindane. These are safer, nonabsorbed insecticides. Crotamiton does, however, have the bonus of relieving itching as it kills mites, whereas lindane is just a mite killer.

A scabies patient will do almost anything to relieve the itching. Will, a painter, had an itchy rash for weeks and discovered his own "solution" to the problem. Quite early in the course of his disease he had noticed that he never got the itchy spots on his hands if he cleansed his hands each day with turpentine or mineral spirits. So Will started washing all his itchy areas with turpentine, which quite effectively kept his scabetic infestation down to a minimum. But then he showed up in my office with severe turpentine irritation of his skin. It was only coincidentally that I noticed during the examination of his dry, red, cracked skin that he had some small bumps around his navel and around the head of his penis that looked like classical scabies bumps. Around his navel there were even a few tiny burrows where mites had quite obviously taken up residence. Inspection of his hands, however, revealed no scabies spots there at all. Apparently his "turpentine treatment," while very irritating, was somewhat effective in eradicating the mites.

Seborrheic Keratoses

LIFE'S BARNACLES

These ugly, stuck-on, waxy-looking brown spots, which my chief of dermatology used to call "barnacles on the ship of life," are real nuisances in the elderly. They scale, flake off, and itch horribly in some patients. After I treated my first one, I renamed them as "spots due to wisdom and maturity." One dermatologist calls them "late-onset birthmarks" because the genes necessary to form them have always been there, but the spots don't appear until the necessary age is reached.

The real name for these crusty things is seborrheic keratosis (sebo-REE-ick ker-a-TOE-sis). Classically, their waxy, stuck-on appearance has been likened to a drop of warm brown candle wax on the skin. Often they have little dots on their surfaces, indicating areas where the keratin, or dead layer of the skin, has formed small plugs.

I've seen as many as several hundred of these flaky spots on a single patient. Often, they do itch somewhat. Basically, though, they're harmless "gifts" from your ancestors; that is, they are inherited, and you're quite likely to pass them on to your progeny.

Seborrheic keratoses (SKs) are so widespread in our population that I've received literally hundreds of questions regarding them. In a television interview, I recently offered an informational sheet telling people about seborrheic keratosis, and the next day I received 400 individual inquiries about it. You can see what an incredibly common and annoying problem this is.

Unfortunately, family physicians often say to leave them alone, but only until the doctors themselves get a few. Then they swarm into the offices of their dermatologist colleagues to have them removed. And this is partly understandable. They spend their whole day dealing with serious diseases; often, they don't realize how distressing a disfiguring spot on a person's face, neck, or back can be. And even if they did, they really don't have the tools to fix the spots without scarring.

This brings up the treatment of SKs. Ordinarily, we use cryosurgery (freezing with liquid nitrogen). Light freezing of the spot causes a microscopic blister to form under the keratosis. This dries up into a scablike crust, which falls off within two to three weeks.

Usually, no mark is left when the crusts fall off. Sometimes dark complected patients have a small dark spot left in the area, but this should fade nicely with time. "Just think, Dr. Bark," said one elderly patient with virtually hundreds of SKs, "I'll be able to swim as fast as my kids when you get all these barnacles off!"

Is it possible to scratch them off? Probably not. The cells that make up the hard spot, or keratosis, are in the deep epidermis, and it's unlikely that you could scratch hard enough to remove them for good. However, a modification of "fingernail surgery" has been developed, in which the dermatologist freezes the spots lightly and then scrapes them off with a curved knife blade called a curette.

After this procedure, the patient actually leaves the office without the spot. The disadvantages of this cryocurettage method, as it is called, is that an occasional patient will be more disposed to develop hyperpigmentation, or pigment darkening after cryocurettage than after straight cryosurgery without the scraping procedure. The patient's going to have a scab anyway, so why not let the freezing do the whole job? In addition, bleeding and scarring occur sometimes with the scraping technique.

Do SK's ever turn into skin cancer? Virtually never, assuming that you've got the right diagnosis. However, one of my friends said once, "Assume makes an ASS out of U and ME." So get them checked to make sure of the correct diagnosis. The fact is that seborrheic keratoses are neither sunlight induced nor precancerous, if that is what they are.

Why take them off, then? Seborrheic keratoses slowly enlarge over the years, and even though you may not think that from a cosmetic standpoint they need to come off right now, you may in the future. So I usually advise patients to have the ones in potentially objectionable areas removed when they are small. It certainly makes the task easier. This also prevents cracking and itching in the spots, which can cause you to scratch them and get them infected, causing more of a problem in removal. They should not be CUT off, however, if you're interested in not having a scar in all those areas. Regular cutting surgery goes right through the thickness of the skin, causing a scar every time one of them is taken off. But cryosurgery makes a very "physiological" type of split right at the base of the epidermis, which doesn't scar. As far as scarring is concerned, much the same is true for burning them off, except the smallest of them, called skin tags. If the current is very low in the electric needle, some of these lesions can be coaxed off without scarring, but this takes a very deft hand on the part of the surgeon.

SKs are not contagious. They have, though, in the past, been spoken of as seborrheic "warts," and that's probably where that idea came from. Touching them, or someone who has them, is not going to cause them to appear.

ℐkin Cancer

FRY NOW, PAY LATER*—
SUN CANCERS, MELANOMAS, AND MOLES

Over 600,000 cases of skin cancer happen in this country every year, making it the most common of all types of cancer. Over 30,000 cases of malignant melanoma (the most deadly form of skin cancer) are discovered each year, resulting in over 9,000 deaths. And why is this problem so massive in proportions? Sunlight! It's nearly the sole cause of two major types of skin cancers, and the probable cause in many of the melanoma cases. In fact, studies show that about 68–92 percent of all melanomas worldwide are caused by sunlight. And up to 66 percent of all melanomas would not occur if kids would avoid tanning and other sun exposure during the ages of one to seventeen. Incredible!

But people still love to lie in the sun.

As a child, I was guilty of my own sun indiscretions. I remember a radio contest one year in which we all taped our backs with the call letters of an Akron station. The winner (not me) was the guy who got the greatest contrast between his sizzled back and the baby-white skin below the letters. Nowadays, we dermatologists must contend with much more than a single dark tan. We now have that "wonderful" invention, the tanning salon, to keep the damage coming year round.

TANNING SALONS

How safe are tanning salons? Can they actually be harmful to your skin? Are they worse than the sun? Frankly, going to a tanning salon is an open and frontal assault on your skin. The American Academy of Dermatology, in 1979, issued a general alert concerning the practice. Tanning salon patrons may, through the years, develop many

---

* Used with permission of the American Cancer Society.

more skin cancers because of this intense, direct exposure to the exact wavelengths of light that a person shouldn't have.

Worse than the sun? Certainly! These booths emit the dangerous, cancer-causing rays at a very close distance, giving a much more concentrated exposure than ordinary sunlight.

TANNING BEDS

In response to all the advertisements touting these "tanning beds" as safer, the American Academy of Dermatology's Task Force on Photobiology has issued a release giving their views on the new booths. They can actually cause a host of serious problems, including cataracts, skin cancer, accelerated aging, potentiation of the cancer-causing effects of regular sunlight, and, believe it or not, possibly even changes in the body's immune system.

A patient of mine gave his opinion on those dangers, when, after I explained the complications of tanning beds, he exclaimed, "Wow, you mean they can really cause all that? No wonder they look so much like coffins!"

Stay away from them! Your poor skin has enough to contend with, just with all the sunlight chemicals and natural pollutants, let alone this source of artificial pollutant, which can, in fact, be 1,000 times more damaging than regular sunlight.

SUNLIGHT AND VITAMIN D

You'll get plenty of vitamin D from milk supplementation and other dietary sources without needing sunlight to process it for you. And the sun is definitely not needed for other health reasons. The little bit we all get walking to and from the car is a hundred times more than we need.

A brownish-tanned lady once said to me, "But I always look so healthy when I'm tanned." I was shocked. Beauty, in this regard, is definitely in the eye of the beholder. "I think you look quite damaged, myself," I considered saying to her. Tanning is the first and best indicator that sun damage has already been done to your skin. While the tan protects you somewhat on future exposure to the sun, it can't stop the real damage from building up cumulatively—year after year after wrinkled, cancerous year!

SUNLIGHT AND THE SKIN

In the old days of bonnets and parasols, women would have cursed every minute they were forced to be in the sun. They seem to have known what it would do to them. But somewhere along the line, women, and men too, forgot about the horrendous things sunlight does to skin. Lately, I've been encouraging everyone to join what I call my "Tan Is Tacky Club," to try to reeducate people about sun damage.

I once watched a movie being filmed in the Arizona desert, and I was amazed at the lengths to which the young, smooth-skinned actresses would go in order not to be in the sunlight. There was a whole crew of men with umbrellas assigned to shield them from the bright sun. After all, those actresses knew that their very careers depended on the avoidance of sun wrinkles. Oh, if we would all realize that fact!

And now, scientists tell us that we must worry much more in future years about the gigantic hole in the ozone layer, about which we all have heard. Frankly, ozone is the only substance that keeps us from sizzling in the sunlight like so many potato chips. It's the wonderful stuff made by lightning that absorbs most of the damaging ultraviolet rays of the sun. Fluorinated hydrocarbon sprays break down the ozone, letting the sun shine in. That's why everyone was anxious to stop them from being used several years ago. Now, almost all the sprays are pressurized with other gases such as isobutane, which are harmless to the ozone layer. Trouble is, not every country is using the nonfluorinated hydrocarbons, so we still have a massive planet-wide problem to deal with in centuries to come.

Unhappily, aerosol sprays are not the only sources of damage to the ozone layer. We've still got a problem with high-flying commercial and military jets that could result in more skin cancers in the future.

SUNLIGHT AND AGING

You bet! Sunlight is the prime cause of the aged look as the years pass. I often use this fact in order to convince patients to protect their skin from sun. It seems as if very few people listen if I say, "You're going to get skin cancer if you don't change your sunbathing habits." But if I tell them, "Sunbathing will make you look like a wrinkled old prune," they'll listen to me almost every time.

So, to accomplish my purpose of shading as much skin as possible, I'll appeal to vanity any time. If it works, use it!

Know how to prove to yourself that sunlight causes the aged look? Take a look at the neck skin of a farmer or a sailor, and then look at the covered chest skin of the same person. The neck skin is wrinkled and coarse, just like football leather, but the covered skin is as smooth as a newborn baby's bottom. And yet that skin's the same age as the wrinkled skin. Are fine, age/sun-induced wrinkles unavoidable? Of course not! There's no reason to count on wrinkles, any more than you'd count on any other personal tragedy (which is what we skin doctors think wrinkles are). If you avoid alcohol, is it likely that you'll still get cirrhosis? If you don't eat like a whale, is it likely you'll get fat? Of course not, and the same holds true for sun damage.

Of course, there are some gravity-type wrinkles that still occur, but they're really minor compared with the intense wrinkling of sun damage.

SUNBATHING AND CANCER

The distribution of skin cancers on the human body ought to tell you what causes it. The vast majority of skin cancers occur on sun-exposed skin. If you could spend just one day with me in my office, you'd be convinced of this simple fact forever. If you could just see how many faces and noses skin cancer surgeons have to whittle on to remove skin cancers, you would never doubt it. As one of my associates carved off the tip of the nose of an eighteen year old with skin cancer one day, she whispered tearfully, "I'll not fail to listen to you again!"

It's definitely true that some families tend to get what I prefer to call "sun cancer" a lot more easily and earlier than other families. These are the Scotch-Irish, Nordic, and Scandinavian peoples with blue eyes, fair skin, and red hair. They are at tremendously greater risk than darker-skinned people, but still, dark-skinned Mediterranean types certainly can get skin cancers, and often do. It's just that they are afforded a little more natural protection in the form of melanin skin pigmentation.

OLDER SUNBATHERS

If a woman of fifty-five years of age has been sunbathing all her life, can she still sunbathe without damaging her skin? That damage she's been incurring all these years has never left her. It's cumulative, that is, it builds up over a person's entire lifetime, just like X-ray therapy. Every sun-exposed skin cell carries the genetic damage of each and every exposure. I wish it did go away. Then the number of skin cancers would actually get less with old age, assuming we could finally convince the public to refrain from sunbathing.

But take hope! The cellular sun damage won't fade with time, but your wrinkles might. Researchers have discovered that the sun damage to the dermis, which is responsible for all the fine wrinkles of old age, does indeed lessen with age, if the skin is no longer exposed. To prove this, they've done some rather bizarre tests. They've applied sunscreens to one half of the body of elderly nursing home patients, and rolled them out into the sun day after day. With enough time, biopsy specimens from the skin of the sunscreened side did show reversal of the changes leading to wrinkling. It certainly pays to avoid the sun!

I've often been asked, usually right after explaining the damage of sunbathing, when's the best time to lie out in the sun? My favorite reply is: About 11:30 at night! Really there's no good time to destroy your skin. We do know that the worst times are from 10 A.M. to 2 P.M. And, of course, the sun's much hotter in southern climes, because, due to the earth's curvature, you're lying physically closer to the sun. In tropical areas one can get "cutaneously cooked" and "dermally done" in just a matter of minutes.

SUNLIGHT THROUGH WINDOW GLASS

Many people complain that there is one place where they are legitimately and frequently in the sun. Usually this is when they are in their cars—the sun is extremely intense through the windows. But I've got great news for you. Sunlight through window glass is completely harmless! The damaging part, called UVB, is filtered out as the light strikes the glass. Its energy is transformed into great amounts of radiant heat, which streams into the car. That's why the interior temperature of a car can reach 120 to 130° F quite easily, on just a moderately warm day. It can become a veritable solar furnace in there. (No wonder so many animals die when left in cars.)

Now think of this. That terrific energy would have been available to damage and irrevocably alter the genetic material of your skin cells had you been directly exposed. That's even one more fact which should convince you to stay out of the sun's direct rays.

COSMETICS AND SKIN CANCER

I have often been asked if there is any connection between skin cosmetics and cancer. Indeed there is! The first prevents the second. For instance, because they wear lipstick, women have an almost negligible incidence of lip cancer. It stops the harmful, cancer-causing rays of the sun from striking the lips. The same can be true for the rest of the face, especially if one of the newer, sunscreen-containing cosmetics is used.

ITCHING AND OTHER SKIN CANCER SIGNS

Itching has been discovered to be one of the cardinal signs of skin cancer.

Have your dermatologist check your skin spot if it:

1. Itches.
2. Changes in color.
3. Bleeds.
4. Won't heal.
5. Forms a scar for which there was no injury.
6. Turns red, white, blue, or black.
7. Develops a surrounding halo of whiteness.
8. Has uneven pigment or notches in the pigment's edges.
9. Ulcerates or erodes.

You should examine your entire skin surface once yearly for any spots that display any of these signs. If you've got any of these signs of skin cancer, run, don't walk, to your dermatologist for a checkup.

Itching in skin cancers has always been somewhat of a mystery. We're just now starting to figure out why it happens. Itching is one of the few ways that skin has of calling attention to itself when something is wrong. In fact, itching may be caused by the body's immune system. If the immune system detects changes in cells that make those cells look foreign, as cancer cells would, for instance, it calls out various destroyer cells to try to eliminate the invaders. It often does this successfully, too. There are noted cases of virtual resolution of cancers, including skin cancers, that look like "miracle cures" because of the effective surveillance of the immune system. Researchers think, in fact, that each person develops many cancers over a lifetime and that the immune system wipes them out very effectively.

So itching should be a cardinal signal that something has gone wrong in the skin. Heed the signal. You may get only one chance.

How does a physician know that a spot is okay by just looking at and examining it? This question reminds me of the fifties' joke about the violinist who stops a Beatnik on a New York street corner and asks, "Hey, buddy, how do I get to Carnegie Hall?"

"Practice, man, practice!" the Beatnik answers.

It takes a lot of learning and practice to make the judgment calls on tens and tens of lesions every day. I guess that's why it takes so long to become a dermatologist.

SUNSPOTS (ACTINIC KERATOSES)

Have you seen spots on your skin that are rough and scale off, smooth over for a while, and then repeat this cycle? These spots and others like them may be actinic keratosis (AK). This is usually a reddish, slightly scaly spot on a light-exposed area of the skin. They begin somewhat brown in color, progress to red, and then get slightly to moderately scaly. The importance of actinic keratoses is that they can turn into skin cancers, and often do. Experts feel as many as 10 percent of AKs will, sooner or later, turn into skin cancers, usually of the squamous cell type (more about this later).

Actinic keratoses do scale off from time to time, and in fact, that's what may keep people from getting them treated earlier. They think that since their spot peeled off once or twice before, it'll keep peeling off in layers until it's all gone. Usually, this is untrue, because no matter how many times the spot peels off, the underlying cells that make the scaly part remain to remake the scale.

However, as much as I hate to say it, picking them off doesn't really make them any worse. More than one dermatologist feels that shaving is responsible for the very few AKs we see on the cheeks of men, while the foreheads, bald spots, ears, neck, and hands are often covered with them. I'm not advising you to try to pick off your premalignant lesions, however. Get them checked!

In my office, AKs are usually removed by cryosurgery—spraying on liquid nitrogen to freeze them and make them peel off. The process stings a little, but usually leaves no sign that the AK was ever there. Cryosurgery is extremely useful for a limited number of lesions and usually eliminates them permanently in the areas sprayed.

If, however, we take the example of actinic keratoses on the face, the entire face was exposed for years to about the same amount of light, so that in areas that were not frozen, we could expect new lesions to arise with time. This is called the "field theory" in dermatology, indicating that the lesions can arise anywhere in the field that has received the damage (in this case, from the sun).

AK is not really the same as a senile keratosis. A senile keratosis is a seborrheic keratosis. These are not premalignant. Constant rubbing of a spot used to be thought to cause cancer. It does not. What it does cause is irritation, which can result in a lot of confusion and anxiety when the spot is seen by a physician. If you'll remember, redness, scaling, bleeding, and so on are all signs of skin cancer, and that's also how doctors tell if a spot's malignant or not. Therefore, if a place is constantly irritated by clothing, a physician might look at the spot and think it's a skin cancer, when, in fact, it's not. This may prompt the doctor to take off a much larger piece of skin than necessary as a precaution, in case it's proven to be a skin cancer. Understand? I hope so. Anyway, the bottom line is that the spot should probably be removed so that it doesn't confuse the picture if it ever does get irritated.

EFUDEX—THE TMB
(TOO MANY BIRTHDAYS) CREAM

TMBs are marks that result from "too many birthdays." Certainly this applies, in a way, to AKs. The cream that best treats many lesions or spots at a time is Efudex. This potent anticancer drug, called 5-fluorouracil, was discovered quite by accident to have destructive effects on premalignant lesions of the skin, namely, actinic keratoses. When the drug was injected into cancer patients, a curious reddening of their sunspots was noticed, and some of the spots actually faded away permanently. Startled, the researchers tried the drug in a topically applied form that also worked spectacularly on AKs. This drug is now marketed under the brand name Efudex.

The substance will not treat all TMBs, however, and it's a pretty tough treatment program to go through. You see, Efudex works not only on the scaly lesions you can see, but also on the microscopic ones you don't even know are there yet. So patients on Efudex therapy start to get red in all sorts of places they never even suspected they had sunspots before. And the redness, while tolerable, does often get quite severe. The treatment has to be continued for three to six weeks in order to knock out all the premalignant lesions. It's tough to find patients willing to go through the redness and scabbing of this course of therapy, because almost everyone turns out to have three family reunions, an audience with the Pope, and an appearance on *Good Morning America* scheduled during the proposed treatment period! If the treatment is stopped too early, only a fraction of the lesions will be wiped out.

Sunlight makes the Efudex reaction much more severe and irritating, so most patients are cautioned to perform this treatment only in the wintertime, when their sun exposure could be expected to be at a minimum. That makes it even tougher for those who would like to leave town on vacation while their faces are red from the medicine—they can't go to a sunny area.

As with all medicines, an allergy can develop to Efudex. When this happens, swelling, redness, and blisters are seen in the normally shaded areas. This is a true contact allergy, and will probably prohibit the use of Efudex in such a case. Your dermatologist can tell you how to do a patch test or a use test in order to see if you're allergic or not.

A new cream called Actinex is detailed to wipe out these pre-malignant sunspots, as does Efudex, but in our hands, this cream not only does not seem to do a thorough enough job of eliminating the spots, but also has a frequent incidence of topical allergy, resulting in blisters and facial swelling. I have ceased using this drug and have returned to the time-honored gold standard drug, Efudex.

BASAL CELL CARCINOMA— THE MOST COMMON CANCER

Basal cell carcinomas (BCCs) are the most common type of cancer. There are 600,000 of these spots that occur in this country every year.

BCCs are slow-growing, indolent tumors that don't usually spread to internal organs. They begin as small, flesh-colored, whitish, or even slightly red bumps on the skin. They very often are discrete, isolated bumps, but occasionally take on a diffuse appearance that's much more difficult to eradicate. This particular form is called the morphea, or diffuse-type, BCC. The bumplike BCCs are called nodular basal cells. Often they will ulcerate and bleed, forming recurrent crusts. This is the classic sign the American Cancer Society tells us about in their warning, "Beware of a sore that doesn't heal!"

Bleeding is usual for BCCs because of the many tiny blood vessels that develop over the surface of these tumors. They can be seen quite easily on close inspection of a BCC with a hand magnifying lens.

Some BCCs look like depressed areas in the skin, often surrounded by a tiny raised border. Occasional ones even have a "chewed-out" appearance that the very descriptive early dermatologists called "rodent ulcers," after their resemblance to the ragged, punched-out border of a rat bite.

Almost universally caused by sunlight, BCCs are dangerous because they expand locally and invade, by direct extension, adjacent structures. This becomes a matter of serious concern when these lesions are located next to important structures such as the nose, eyes, and ears.

BCCs are removed in much the same ways as are SCCAs (squamous cell carcinoma). In the elderly, and in persons who would not be expected to tolerate surgery very well, radiation therapy can be used adequately.

What if a basal cell carcinoma was removed years ago and has recurred? The most effective method for removal of a recurrent skin cancer is a relatively new surgical technique: Mohs microscopically controlled excision. Mohs surgery involves the exact mapping of the tumor. The lesion is cut off in horizontal sections, each of which is labeled and processed for immediate examination. If any of the sections still have skin cancer in them, then just a little more adjacent skin in that area is cut out again. This is repeated until all the sections submitted are tumor-free.

Mohs surgery results in the highest possible cure rate for BCCs and SCCAs. For first-time-treated tumors in difficult areas of the skin, such as near the nose, eyes, ears, or other important structures, it is appropriate primary therapy, although it's considerably more complicated and more expensive than conventional surgery. Also, it's not available everywhere, so your dermatologist will discuss its need and availability in your case.

SQUAMOUS CELL SKIN CANCER

Squamous cell carcinoma (SCCA) is the second most common type of skin cancer dermatologists treat. It's caused by continuous sun damage to the mid- and upper epidermis, or topmost skin layer. These lesions are important because they are the ones that result directly from AKs. They grow by local extension and usually do not spread through the lymphatic drainage system, or the blood vessel network. In other words, for most types of SCCAs, local surgical removal will take care of them.

Squamous cancers look like thickened AKs. That is, they frequently have the redness and scaliness of actinic keratoses, but they look more aggressive, with more redness, more scale, and occasionally crusting and bleeding. Usually, they are thick enough to have a harder, or indurated, feel. Squamous cancers usually are not accompanied by the blackish pigment we often see in melanomas, but they can be various shades of brown or brown-red.

Interestingly, the first draft of this part of this book did not contain the above description. I omitted it because I felt that words could not adequately describe what it takes us dermatologists three years to spot and identify accurately. I still believe, even after adding the above information, that you should not try to diagnose your own skin cancers. These morphological signs of skin cancer are added so that you will have any suspicious spot checked without delay. So use the signs I list here, but use them as a guide to alert you to see your dermatologist. He or she has the experiential equipment to diagnose your problem.

While the treatment for SCCA is surgical removal, this can include several types of surgery. The first and probably most common type is standard knife removal, in which the spot is cut out and the edges of the remaining wound are stitched shut. This effective method results in a linear, or linelike, scar.

The second method is by what we call the shave, curettage, and electrodesiccation (C&ED) method. In this technique, the lesion is numbed with a local anesthetic and shaved off tangential to the skin, and the site of the cancer is scraped vigorously with a curved knife blade called a curette. (The shaved-off part of the tumor is sent off to the pathologist to confirm its type.) The curette scrapes away any remaining tumor. This scraping procedure is performed on each of three different surgical planes, or levels, and after each of the scrapings, the site of the cancer is thoroughly buzzed with an electric needle to assure that a few more cell layers are killed off each time. This gives a higher cure rate for the procedure. In fact, the 90 to 94 percent cure rate of this so-called C&ED procedure is equal to that of the knife-removal technique. This is the type of procedure President Reagan had done on his nose in 1985 for a basal cell cancer.

The third method for removing this type of skin cancer is cryosurgery. A superstrong freeze is delivered to the tumor, which kills off the cancer cells. As you might guess, this type of freeze is much deeper than that used to, say, freeze a wart or a seborrheic keratosis. Often, a thermocouple (an implanted thermometer in a needle) is used to monitor the depth of freeze to assure the best treatment of the cancer. It's a detailed procedure, and it results in a fairly severe blister that weeps for a few days, crusts over, and then falls off in four to six weeks.

The scars left from the second and third methods are disk-shaped and usually somewhat whiter than the surrounding skin. But the methods do provide a good cure rate with as little defect as possible. Many of us use the cryosurgical and C&ED methods for most of the skin cancers we see in the office.

If you should happen to have an SCCA on your lip, that's a different story. This particular type of squamous cancer does occasionally spread to other areas of the body, so it's absolutely critical to get it removed as soon as possible. There is, however, another condition, called actinic cheilitis (pronounced kigh-LIGHT-is), which is chronic inflammation of the lip due to sun damage. It's the lip equivalent of an actinic keratosis (AK).

Shield your lips with Eclipse Lip Protectant or Chap Stick 15 SPF lip balm so that the damage does not occur.

Actinic cheilitis may be treated, after biopsy confirmation that no cancer is yet present, by cryosurgery or by Efudex applications. Either one will temporarily cause a sore lip, but it's worth it to get a potentially fatal condition resolved.

For a comparison of basal and squamous skin cancers, see the following table.

If you have a case of fairly severe actinic cheilitis, your doctor wants to make sure that all those bad cells get taken care of. For this, they sometimes use a procedure called a "lip shave." He or she will remove the skin on your lower lip (shaved), so that all the damaged skin is gone. After the shaving off of all the damaged tissue, the soft, moist mucous membrane inside the lip is pulled outward, or "advanced," to form a new, normal-looking lip line. This procedure's marvelous. It relieves you of all your scaliness and premalignant lip spots all at once.

The lip usually heals up beautifully with almost no sign of any previous damage. But remember that the same damage can recur if you again get a lot of sunlight exposure. And the second time around, it's not as easy to find good tissue for the lip shave procedure.

MELANOMA—TIMING IS CRITICAL

While all skin cancers are important, not all are immediately life threatening. For instance, the basal cell carcinoma and squamous cell carcinomas we've discussed often take months to years even to become noticeable, and many more years to become life threaten-

CHARACTERISTICS OF BASAL AND SQUAMOUS SKIN CANCERS

	BASAL	*SQUAMOUS*
Nodule (raised bump)	Frequent	Occasional
Tiny blood vessels on	Frequent	Rare surface
Scaling	Less common	Frequent
Color	Pale, pearly, rarely pigmented	Red or red-brown
Internal spread	Extremely rare	Very rare
Sun-caused	Yes	Yes
Treatment	Varies, multiple	Varies, multiple
Prognosis	Excellent	Excellent
Growth pattern	Slow	Slow
Invades local structures	Yes	Yes
Preceded by actinic keratosis (AK)	No	Yes, usually
Seen in old burn scars	Rarely	Yes, occasionally
Location	Light-exposed areas	Light-exposed areas
"Rodent ulcer"	Often	Rarely
Bleeding	Yes	Less frequently

ing (the exception to this, obviously, is the tumor that is located near a vital structure, such as a tear duct, ear canal, or eyelid).

But melanoma is a different story. This tumor of pigment cells is life threatening, by definition, if it exists. Except for certain rare instances of regression of melanoma, all melanomas, if left untreated, have the potential to cause the demise of the patient.

Melanoma starts as a collection of just a few pigment cells that multiply in a disorganized fashion. When they are first noticeable, the tiny spot they form is quite thin. It thickens as it grows, pressing deeper and deeper into the dermis below and actually growing into it.

The flat spot thickens progressively into a small lump (nodule). The thicker the lesion (pathologists actually measure every malignant melanoma, or MM, with a microscopic ruler), the worse the outlook for cure. All MMs have the potential of spreading in three ways: They may grow directly into surrounding structures (direct invasion); they may spread via the lymph system (lymphatic spread); or they may spread through the bloodstream (hematogenous spread). All forms of spread are called metastases. Metastases of MM may occur at any time, but are much less likely if the tumor is removed when it's still thin.

"Melanoma" is a word that is derived from the word "melanin." That's the pigmentary material that is responsible for all the various shadings of color in human skin. The melanin is made by special cells called melanocytes, which are hidden deep in the base of the uppermost skin layer, the epidermis. While melanocytes ordinarily go about their normal factory-like production of melanin, they can occasionally start to multiply in a greatly disorganized fashion. The tumor that results is the MM.

The crucial fact to remember in melanomas, however, is that timing is ultracritical. If you have any of the symptoms of skin cancers we've discussed, please make the investment in this book count and get your dermatologist to check out the suspicious spots. If you have a suspicious spot of any kind, I cannot tell you anything more important than to go see a dermatologist immediately. You may have a malignant melanoma. If you catch it early, it can be readily cured. If you wait, however, you could be in very bad trouble.

The exact causes of melanoma are still a mystery. Apparently there's some disordering of the skin cells' normal multiplication, but what turns on this disorder, or, rather, what cancels out the ordinarily magnificent orderliness with which these cells multiply, is unknown.

However, we're now getting some hints. Melanomas show a surprisingly high occurrence rate on sun-exposed skin, a disturbing fact that is just now becoming apparent. Heretofore, we thought all we really had to worry about because of sun exposure were wrinkles, basal cell carcinomas, and squamous cell carcinomas.

But as the ozone layer decreases further and further, and as the quest for the "great American tan" continues, the incidence of MM has reached over 30,000 new cases each year, with about 9,000 deaths yearly from the disease. So we're getting quite a bit more vocal about the deleterious effects of sunshine.

BLUE NEVUS

Not every dark spot on the skin is a melanoma. Some spots are very dark, and seem to have lighter-colored skin over them. While it's very possible that such a dark spot could be an MM, it's possible that it is a benign lesion called a blue nevus. That's a noncancerous blue-black nodule deep under the skin, the look of which is generally calmer than that of an MM. Also, they don't grow, scab over, crust, bleed, change color, or itch, as BCCs, SCCAs, and MMs do. But because of the pigment, which is apparently deep down in the skin, I would biopsy such a spot every time.

If it were discovered on pathology exam that the lesion does indeed turn out to be a benign blue nevus, at least it will be off, and the patient need not have to worry about it anymore.

COLORS IN MELANOMAS

Melanomas come in many different colors. They may be tan, brownish, brown-black, blue-black, black, or even completely colorless without any pigment at all. As they grow, they may have a deep blue shade, indicating pigment deep down in the dermis, or they may be reddish, indicating inflammation (the body's reaction against the tumor), or even white in some areas, indicating regression and resolution of a part of the growth. The histological type (what it looks like to the pathologist), depth, and thickness are far more important than the color of the tumor. We'll discuss more about thickness and prognosis elsewhere. Melanomas are somewhat more common in fair-skinned, blue-eyed, red- and blond-haired, Scotch-Irish, English, and Nordic individuals because of their increased sensitivity to damaging sunlight. Kids should definitely take that into consideration when they think about achieving the Great American Tan! Anyone, however, can get melanoma, so any suspicious spots should be checked no matter what the age or color of the person.

Dysplastic Nevus Syndrome

More important, though, is the question about a possible genetic tendency toward MM. There have been some important findings about a special hereditary form of MM. Since 1952, sporadic cases of a condition called dysplastic nevus syndrome (DNS) have been found. This is apparently a dominant hereditary characteristic, afflicting several members in a family with strange-looking moles and cutting across generations. As a result of this condition, these individuals have a much higher probability of getting MM. That's good enough reason why every person on this planet should have at least one "mole check," as we call it in our office, most urgently in his or her childhood. If it is discovered that a person has DNS, very close follow-up by the dermatologist is recommended, possibly as often as every six months or so.

Dysplastic nevi are those moles that exhibit strange pigmentary findings when the dermatologist sees them. Often they are quite small, but more often they are larger and are seen in multiple areas of the body. The back and chest are the most common areas, but legs and scalp can have these lesions too. In fact, any area can.

The moles look strange because they have diffuse pigment in them, which is as if someone put a blob of brown pigment onto the skin and then smeared it into the surrounding skin. That is, they are smudgy around the edges. Often they have a little bit of darker pigment in the center, a fact that leads dermatologists to look for this so-called, "fried egg sign."

MOLES (NEVI)

Many patients and their relatives ask about the differences between a wart and a mole. The following chart will tell you the principal differences. But if you have any doubt, see your dermatologist!

Many moles contain hairs that project from their surfaces. Moles form deep down in the skin, at the level of the formation of the hair follicles. The dark hairs and the moles develop together. I've had many patients come into the office complaining that they are tired of clipping off the hairs over their moles.

CHARACTERISTICS OF WARTS, MOLES, AND MELANOMAS

CHARACTERISTIC	WART	MOLE	MELANOMA
Color	Pale, skin-colored	Varied (pale, tan, brown, black)	Brown-black + red, white, or blue
Surface	Rough	Smooth to bumpy	Smooth to crusted and bleeding
Border	Even	Mostly even to uneven	Irregular, notched
Grouped	Yes, often	Very rarely	No
Infectious	Yes, virus-caused	No	No
Genetic predisposition	No	Yes	Occasionally
Malignant potential	None or very rare	Occasional but rarely	These *are* malignant
Location	Hands, feet most common	Chest, back, face, scalp most common	Anywhere
Blackened surface capillaries	Yes	No	No, but may bleed intermittently
Congenital (present at birth)	No	Occasional	Rarely
Influenced by sunburns	No	No	Yes

"Why aren't you just plucking them out?" I usually ask.

"Why, Dr. Bark," they ask agitatedly, "didn't you know that'll cause skin cancer in them?"

"As a matter of fact, I didn't! Where'd you hear that, anyway?"

"My Granny said a relative of her aunt's mother pulled a hair out of a black mole and she died of cancer."

"Hmmm. Sounds like really accurate firsthand information, doesn't it? Just remember that you can believe only 50 percent of what you read, and 0 percent of what you hear, okay?"

The fact is that these hairs have nothing to do with the malignant potential of moles. Moles are just collections of pigment-containing cells, and they have no more tendency to turn into skin cancers than any pigment cell anywhere in the body—and there are millions of them. The majority of melanoma skin cancers (the "deadly" type) arise *de novo*, i.e., in spots where absolutely no mole ever existed. Other melanomas, which the patient thinks arose from a mole, were already skin cancer from day one. But their slow growth in one location makes them look as though they were originally just moles. So go ahead and pull all the hairs out of your moles if you wish.

Patients always want to know about the effect of irritation on moles. In short, it's not likely to produce a skin cancer that wasn't there already, but the fact that you tend to scrape this one off in your daily activities may mean that you should, in fact, consider having it removed to avert this concern in the future. I would.

Most dermatologists remove moles by the shave biopsy technique. In this method of removal, the mole is anesthetized with a tiny drop of numbing medicine. This allows a painless procedure without distortion of the mole's surface. Then the mole is removed so that it is level with the surrounding skin. It's called a "shave biopsy" as opposed to an incisional biopsy, in which the lesion is cut full thickness out of the skin. In most cases, the incisional biopsy needs sutures, whereas the shave biopsy does not. Scarring and healing time are usually minimal with the shave technique. A nice smooth result is usually obtained in this manner. Note that moles are, for the most part, located deep down in the dermis, and therefore, for most moles, only the major fraction is removed by this technique. But it's enough to get a flat-looking spot where there used to be a bump, and a diagnosis is obtained on the biopsy specimen so obtained.

In the old days, doctors used to burn moles off with electric needles, or just cut them off and throw them away. These methods are definitely to be condemned, because they don't allow for the sending off of the specimen to be checked by a pathologist for any possible signs of skin cancer. Make sure that anything removed from your body is sent to a pathologist for examination. Otherwise, you can never know the exact kinds of cells that made up your mole.

The hair exactly over your mole will be removed for the shave biopsy procedure, but it grows back rapidly. Your dermatologist will tell you that since, in this method of removal, there are often some mole cells left, there is at least some chance that the mole could regrow, causing a new molelike bump that may need to be retreated.

Some moles develop whitish halos around themselves. This is a fairly classic description of a mole called Sutton's nevus, or halo nevus. This strange reaction in a mole is just one more way that the body's fabulous immune system is able to patrol for problems inside our bodies. It's apparent that some change is occurring inside the mole that has prompted the immune system to send out the body's defenses to wipe out the problem area. Many dermatologists feel these halo nevi are the precursors to true melanomas, the deadly pigmented skin cancers. Often, melanoma patients will develop halos around their normal moles, which can mean that they are fighting off their melanoma with greater success.

While most of us do shave biopsy these halo nevi, I have never yet seen a melanoma develop in one. So maybe the changes are so early as to be indistinguishable under the pathologist's microscope. Some clinicians choose just to watch these moles, but, following the golden rule, I can only say that I'd want my own Sutton's nevus off if I developed one, so I can do no less for my patients.

Proof that this halo represents the elimination of the mole comes from patients with just the halo, having no mole left whatsoever. They'll often say that they've noticed the disappearance of a large mole that was there several months ago. Strange! And sometimes, the pigment returns to its normal color.

What if you've got a growing mole that changes coloration or itches? Get it off yesterday! You've already got three of the cardinal signs of skin cancer: pigmentary change, growth change, and, most important, itching. Even though soft, fleshy moles seldom, if ever, turn into skin cancer, the fact is that if it is a cancer, the statistics are 100 percent in your case. Can you afford to take that chance? Absolutely not!

There's plenty of ongoing research about moles, but most of it has been centered not on their cause (which is assumed to be genetic) but on their accidental relationship to skin cancers, which I've already discussed.

There appears to be very little probability that lasers will be used for the primary removal of moles. Lasers cut with a beam of light that is at least as hot as the sun, and this intense burning precludes the proper analysis of the cells of the specimen to be removed, by far the most important thing in removing your mole.

Too many people have a propensity to self-treat skin diseases for far too long. If you treat a spot with an over-the-counter medicine and it doesn't clear promptly, you must have it checked.

WHAT TO DO IF YOU SUSPECT SKIN CANCER

Let's take the case of Ron, one of my patients, who complained, "My problem is eczema. I have an embarrassing red mark the size of a penny on my arm, plus a couple of other inconspicuous marks. They don't bother me, but they sure don't look very nice. My doctor tells me there is nothing that can be done for them. Is this true?"

"Probably not," I said. Ron's question is important, though, because of the mistaken assumption that his skin problem is eczema. This happens so often in dermatology that it's frankly tragic. Patients should not be diagnosing problems; they should just be spotting them. That is, you really don't have the training to tell the exact nature of most skin lesions. If Ron's assumption that he has eczema is wrong, he could die for the mistake! Just remember that any scaly spot that stays in one place could be a premalignant or malignant lesion. In good conscience, all such spots must be checked. Don't forget, the person who plays doctor and "treats himself has a fool for a patient!"

How about the doctor who said nothing could be done? Unfortunately, while all dermatologists are doctors, the reverse is not true. One cannot be expected to know every form of therapy for every possible skin disease, plus all the facts necessary to be a general medical doctor, too. We only hope that books like this can aid the lay public and help the individual fill in the gaps in some way.

The Skin Cancer Foundation now advises that a dermatologist screen every immediate blood relative of melanoma patients in order to spot these DNS lesions more rapidly and to take action at a time when it can really help.

SURVIVAL IN MELANOMA

Long-term survival depends largely on the type, depth, and height of your particular MM. There are several different types, all of which have a different prognosis (expected survival time). The most common type we're seeing these days is the very thin MM, which carries with it the best of all possible prognoses.

For instance, very thin MMs (those with a thickness of less than 0.76 millimeter) have an almost 100 percent survival rate. However, the prognosis for thick lesions that have penetrated the fat below the skin is dismal. This is the reason why finding MMs early is so very important.

SUNSCREENS—THE MODERN WAY TO PROTECT

Sunscreens come in two major types. We're all familiar with the old parasol-and-bonnet concept. That's all our ancestors had to prevent themselves from wrinkling up like prunes in the hot sun. This type of sunscreen is the physical type. It includes long sleeves, and white, reflective clothing to shield the tender skin below.

More recently, a new concept in sun protection has evolved with "parasols in a bottle," or chemical sunscreens. These agents are some of the most remarkable chemicals in human history. They are composed of molecules with a special affinity for sunlight. The thin, protective layer they put down can shield you from 99 percent of the sun's harmful rays, depending on the composition of the chemical sunscreen.

What's the best one? You know how to find the best of anything medical? Ask your doctor which one he or she uses. Solbar 50 or Durascreen 30 are the ones I use. The numbers (called sun protection factors, or SPFs) that follow the name of the preparation indicate how much they shield you from the sun. For instance, with no sunscreen at all, the human skin rates a 1. That is, the skin burns in a set number of minutes (the first time) for each person. Now, if that same person, who burns, say, in ten minutes on the year's first exposure, wears a number "8" sunscreening lotion, then he or she would have to stay out for 80 (10 X 8) minutes to get the same degree of burn. In other words, the higher the SPF number, the higher the degree of protection.

The sunscreen manufacturers tell us that each person has to make up his or her own mind regarding the extent of protection needed. We are left to shift for ourselves in determining the amount of damage we want to risk!

I personally believe that all people should give themselves the best possible shot at making it through life "skin cancerless." So use a 30-rated (at least) sunscreen every time you'll get significant sun exposure. You might as well take good care of that skin of yours. It may be the only one you'll ever get!

SWIMMERS, LISTEN UP!

Waterproof sunscreens are getting more and more common. And they work! First, apply the liquid, cream, or spray sunscreens about an hour before you'll expect to be in the water, and again about a half hour before exposure. That'll give your sunscreen a chance to soak right into the dead layer of the skin, called the stratum corneum. That's the important layer that shields us from the various hazards of our environment.

GET SUNGLASSES—BIG ONES!

If you want to protect the skin around your eyes and eyelids, get the biggest sunglasses you're comfortable wearing. My favorites are Fisherman's Sunglasses, from the Orvis Company. They're polarized, with eye protection shields above and at the sides of the eyes. The Noir sunglasses, built originally for skiers and for patients who must undergo powerful light therapy for psoriasis, are good too. You can get them through:

Elder Pharmaceuticals, Inc.
3300 Hyland Avenue
Costa Mesa, CA 92626

YOUR LIPS

Last, and possibly most important, are your lips. Nothing takes the punishment of lips in the sun. The sun damage can be largely prevented, as I've previously stated, by wearing a stick form of sunscreen, such as Chap Stick 15-rated Lip Balm. Another great one is Neutrogena lip protectant.

HATS AND SUN DAMAGE

A hat goes a long way toward preserving your beautiful unwrinkled complexion, but reflected sun is also a real culprit. As much as 90 percent of the incident sunlight on sand can come shooting right back in your face. There's even more reflectance around water. Even grass reflects about 18 percent of the light that strikes it. So don't expect your hat to do it all. Use a sunscreening lotion as well. If you want to get someone you love a really effective sunscreening hat, the one we dermatologists love most is the Tilley Hat. It's a wide-brimmed light-proof hat that *really* protects the face and neck from sun damage. Here's the address:

Tilley Endurables Corp.
3525 Seneca St.
West Seneca, NY 14224

PABA ALLERGY

The most common allergy to sunscreen products is, unfortunately, to the most effective ingredient, PABA. When this allergy occurs, the light-exposed areas break out in a rash of small bumps that itch like crazy. Without treatment, they last for days, and then fade slowly.

It's a tough problem, because PABA is so effective. However, the makers of sunscreens have come up with non-PABA-containing lotions, such as the new Solbar PF. This sunscreen should work wonders for those who couldn't wear sunscreens previously, because of allergies.

Tanning Pills, Lotions, and Stains

The class of drugs called psoralens are terrific photosensitizers—that is, they induce a much exaggerated response to sunlight. Tanning with Oxsoralen (produced from certain plants) occurs very quickly and with much deeper color. Psoralens are capable of inducing severe sunburns, however, and have done this to unwary sunbathers. While Oxsoralen is extremely effective in clearing psoriasis, the risk of severe burns, eye problems, skin cancers, and other difficulties is sufficient enough to keep me from ever using it for routine tanning, except in the worst of skin-disease-affected patients.

In general, though, quick-tanning products such as the plethora of agents sold by cosmetic companies are safe, although I've seen an occasional allergic reaction to them. If you get any rashes while using them, just keep the products in mind as possible causes. Dihydroxyacetone, which is a form of dye, is the major substance in most quick-tanning products, and is known to be a substance that "tans without the sun."

Skin Tags

GIVING THE DEATH PENALTY
TO SKIN TAGS

Small "string moles," or skin tags, as they are called, are made up of two different types of structures. One is a miniature SK, which we've discussed. The other is a tiny outpouching of actual skin, called an acrochordon. String moles are a genetic condition and are more common in those who are overweight.

These lesions are noncontagious and nonmalignant, but they surely are one of the most annoying nuisances of the human skin. They constantly catch on dresses, sweaters, clothing, and necklaces. They're also a favorite target for babies, who'll grab anything in sight and try to twist them off. Ouch! That hurts!

Other favorite places for skin tags to develop are in the armpits and the groin, where they tend to be somewhat bigger. These lesions definitely tend to be more numerous in people who are overweight. It seems, sometimes, that one needs not only the genes for them but the size as well.

Some time ago, researchers reported that skin tags were more likely to occur in diabetics, but the studies necessary to confirm this were apparently never done. It's very possible that, since they occur more often in the overweight individual, obesity is the reason we see more diabetes, too. In other words, obesity may be the cause of both conditions. Recently, a study related them to polyps in the colon as well. So people with bowel symptoms and extremely numerous skin tags should be examined for these large-bowel outgrowths too.

The best treatment is very gentle, delicate electrocution of the string mole with an electric needle. The current must be extremely low in order not to scar the skin underlying the skin tag.

Some patients report that they have taglike lesions on their eyelids. In these cases, a dermatologist should at least evaluate the lesion before anything is done, to make absolutely sure it's just a skin tag. There are virtually hundreds of lumps and bumps that can occur around the eyelids, and proper diagnosis is crucial. However, skin tags, or papillomas, as the eye surgeons (ophthalmologists) call them, are the most common by far.

If, indeed, it is a skin tag, then sparking the spot with an electric needle (again, on very low current) is a logical way to take it off. The largest one of these papillomas, of which I have photos in my collection, was as big as a large grape, on the lower eyelid of one of my patients. It had been there so many years that it had begun to evert, or turn down, the lower lid, so that his eye watered constantly. The tears finally made him seek treatment.

I froze the main body of this huge bump on two different occasions, sparked off the rest with my trusty Electrocator, and he went home happy.

Many patients ask if they are viral bumps, or if rubbing them makes them worse. Do they go away after menopause? This shows the depth of the misinformation on common problems like skin tags. That's exactly why I'm sitting here, slaving over a hot word processor to correct all these crazy myths! Virus? Rubbish! Go away after menopause? Nonsense! And clothes rubbing the skin, as I've said, can irritate them, but cannot cause them.

The old-timers did have one saying that was at least therapeutically effective: Tie a horse hair around the little critters, and they'll fall off in a week. This method of strangulating the blood supply of skin tags is still used effectively by some. However, I think, as do most dermatologists, that something removed from the skin should always be sent in for examination by a pathologist. Don't try this at home.

Dr. Marsh, my mentor in dermatology, has a favorite saying about the growth of new skin tags. "Joe, treating skin tags is like stamping out roaches," he says. "You kill one and ten come to the funeral!" While killing them off doesn't really make new ones appear, the tendency to have them does continue, and new ones grow constantly.

Spider Veins

In most people (70 percent) spiders are the result of the small amount of natural estrogens in our systems. Circulating estrogen (a female hormone) can, under the right circumstances, activate tiny blood vessels to overgrow, forming a spider.

Women have more spiders than men because of their naturally higher estrogen levels, and these levels soar with pregnancy, causing even more of these little nuisances to form. The lucky women are those whose spots actually go away after parturition.

Cream skin lighteners are worthless in removing these dilated, or expanded, capillaries. In fact, by slowly lightening the normal masking pigment overlying these lesions, one could imagine that they might even get worse.

Spiders are not *broken* capillaries or blood vessels. Blood is actively flowing through them constantly. Can they be removed? Yes. Understanding that these are not "broken" veins, you'll understand a lot better how we dermatologists treat them. Our first line of defense is the electrodesiccator, or electric needle. This fantastically useful machine can gently zap a spider vein with a small charge of electricity, sealing its fate permanently. The procedure stings a little, but it's worth it when you walk out of the office usually with no sign of those nasty little spiders (except possibly a little swelling where the vessel was zapped shut).

However, the human circulation is a marvelous machine. It seems to know where it wants blood to flow and will try hard to redrill a hole in the vessel. Usually this will occur within a few days, but may take as long as a month for the spider to start flowing again. If this happens, you'll have to have another treatment to seal it again.

The newest of the treatments for enlarged blood vessels on the face is the use of laser beams for their destruction. Lasers are used for the destruction of single or several enlarged capillaries on the face. This technique is especially useful for the larger grossly expanded veins on the nose, which often accompany the middle-age acnelike disease called rosacea (see elsewhere in this book). The most valuable use for the laser on the face is for people, usually rosacea victims, with totally red noses. In these cases, the nose can be treated widely with the laser to seal almost all the superficial vessels simultaneously.

A large group of internal diseases, the so-called autoimmune diseases such as lupus erythematosus, scleroderma, and so forth, can cause spiders. The take-home message here is that if you or any member of your family have many vascular spiders, you should be seen by a dermatologist, an internist, or a rheumatologist, a specialist in sorting out these rarer, but important disorders.

Diabetics are no more likely to have enlarged vascular spiders than are the nondiabetic population.

Could a face-lift help a person with a lot of capillaries visible on the face? Let's put it this way—a face-lift would be *okay* to perform on such a face, but it wouldn't necessarily be expected to help much. The number of capillaries on the face shouldn't affect one's possibilities for a face-lift at all. But I certainly wouldn't expect a face-lift to cure the spidery look, either.

LEG SPIDERS—A TOUGHER PROBLEM

Veins on the legs are more a problem to dermatologists than veins in other locations. Maybe it's because of the vast numbers of them on the legs. Obliterating them all seems like an insurmountable task. I think they are technically harder to get rid of on the legs, too.

The problem seems to come from the actual anatomy of the leg veins. They are longer and of larger caliber than those we usually see on the face, so a single zap with the electric needle is a lot less likely to knock out a leg vein. When many tiny shocks are used, small dots may appear sometime thereafter, like tiny tracks left by the procedure.

Can lasers be used on the legs? This is one of the most frequently asked questions in the office of dermatologists. While it is possible to use a laser to obliterate a vein in the leg, due to factors of leg circulation and pigmentation, this is fraught with many hazards in the leg areas. It is a very expensive procedure that is generally not used for the removal of leg veins. But read on for a better way! Again, although lasers indeed can obliterate these vessels, the treatment is far from perfect because of the scarring it leaves. We all had hope, when lasers were introduced, that they would solve some of these horrendous cosmetic problems, but, alas, such is not the case.

SCLEROTHERAPY INJECTION

Injection sclerotherapy is one very promising avenue of treatment for medium-sized leg veins that does work when performed by a dermatologist or a surgeon skilled in the technique. The therapy consists of injecting a tiny quantity of sclerosing solution (several are used) into the vein. Incidentally, the needles used are so small that they are hardly visible, and a magnifying lens usually must be used with them.

The solution irritates the lining cells of the tiny blood vessels so much that the vessel dies and is digested (cleaned up) by the body's natural defenses, the white blood cells. While the technique does work, it takes a tremendously patient patient and a patient doctor. Also, the expense can be considerable, so investigate costs carefully before having your veins treated. Some dermatologists are so proficient at performing these little injections that they set aside whole days to do the procedure for the hordes of women desiring it. If your dermatologist or surgeon doesn't do these injections, you might ask him or her for a referral to one who does.

VARICOSE VEINS OF THE SKIN

One patient told me of a spot on his ear that was blue-black and compressible. When he squeezed on it, it got lighter, a fact that made him think he had a cancer in the skin of his ear. But this description fits that of a spot we call a "venous lake." These bumps are sometimes called varicose (enlarged) veins of the skin. They're not cancer, and they won't turn into cancer. Your dermatologist can remove them with a simple minor surgical procedure. These spots are quite similar to the ones historically called "caviar spots" on the undersurface of the tongue. These buckshotlike bumps get slowly more numerous with age. Most of us will have some of them at some time but they're harmless. Look under your tongue to see if you have them already. It'll give you some idea of how many TMBs you've suffered.

STASIS DERMATITIS—A VEIN PROBLEM, NOT A VAIN PROBLEM

If you have slowed circulation in your legs and have brown, scaly areas, occasional swelling of the legs, and a dusky coloration, your problem is probably stasis dermatitis, or irritated skin due to slowing of the circulation. This is an extremely common rash in men as they age, and also in women who have had previous vein operations.

The scaly, itchy rash begins because of the slowed blood flow to the leg skin, caused by atherosclerosis (hardening of the arteries), past vein problems, chronic heart failure, and so on. It's a troublesome disease, because we haven't yet figured out how to prevent problems in the circulatory system. Usually, we end up treating the disease after it has occurred.

I can't stress enough how much leg elevation means in trying to keep leg skin intact, once stasis dermatitis is discovered. Elevation of the heels to a point slightly higher than the hips, without bending the knees, is the best way to get the blood flowing better in the legs.

If you obtain your support hose on your doctor's prescription, such as T.E.D. or Jobst brands, they will most assuredly help your blood flow better in your legs. I myself wear a special type of men's support dress socks. They're called Jobst Stride Stockings, and you can inquire about these very comfortable socks from:

The Jobst Institute
653 Miami Street
P.O. Box 653
Toledo, OH 43694

However, the conventional support hose that are available in department stores are not very effective because they are not custom-measured. They can't, therefore, help individual problem veins. The Jobst Institute, however, will custom-measure your leg so you'll get the greatest benefit from elastic stockings.

The other treatments used in stasis dermatitis are various creams containing enzymes, cortisones, and/or antibiotics.

The brownish-tan stain in the skin of legs with stasis dermatitis is caused by the deposition of iron in the skin from blood that has leaked out previously. This occurs each time a small injury occurs. It's much the same as the staining we discussed under ecchymoses. Some of the pigment is also melanin, the natural color material of the skin. This component of the dark skin color can lighten over time, but it does indeed take a long time.

LEG ULCERS

Ulcers are the most dreaded complication of stasis dermatitis. They result not only from the inflammation of the skin but from the actual death of a patch of it.

Dealing with leg ulcers is one of the hardest tasks facing the dermatologist. Over the years, a hundred different remedies have been tried. We've used everything from twenty-four-karat gold leaf, to antibiotics, to table sugar packed into the ulcer, to creams, injections, and surgery. Many of these have been successful, and each of them has ardent physician supporters. If necessary, good skin can be grafted from another site to cover the open ulcer.

Regardless of which of the many useful treatments is chosen to heal your leg ulcer, it's important to get it healed. Chronic ulcers are a source of infection not only for the legs but for the rest of the body as well.

Sunburn

There are two common degrees of sunburn. I'll review the treatments of each type.

First-degree burn is that which causes just redness of the skin. It heals spontaneously over a few days, usually with desquamation, that is, the peeling of the upper layer of the epidermis, which is shed after the damage is repaired. It's painful, and the best treatments are topical and internal cortisones, which can calm the stinging and redness quite fast. Aspirin, taken as quickly as possible after you know you're burned, is a great help. Some experts think aspirin is good to take even before you incur the burn, because it's been discovered that aspirin inhibits an inflammation-causing compound called prostaglandin, which seems to cause the redness. Redness results from damage to the tiny skin capillaries, which swell up massively when the sun irritates them. I've seen sunburn so severe that the capillaries have even leaked out tiny dots of blood below the skin.

Second-degree sunburn consists of blisters. It can be a true medical emergency if a large enough area is affected. It's very important to treat this as soon as possible because fluid loss can occur. This can cause weakness and even shock if severe enough.

Treatment includes steroids, both topically and internally, as well as cool soaks, antibiotics, and sometimes even tetanus reimmunization. Every second-degree blistering sunburn should be seen and treated by a doctor.

SUN REACTIONS FROM DRUGS

Some drugs cause the skin to be extremely sensitive to sun exposure. For instance, medicines such as the thiazide diuretics ("water pills"), which are quite commonly used to control high blood pressure and the leg swelling that can result from bad leg circulation and heart failure, can cause a violent stinging, redness, burning, and itchy skin rash.

The next most frequent cause of photodermatitis is soap. Harsh antibacterial soaps can and do quite often cause reaction to the sun. That's because they contain an antibiotic substance that reacts with the sunlight.

Of course, there are many other causes of this sun-stinging reaction, and your dermatologist will undoubtedly take a detailed history to determine the exact cause.

Sun Spots in Teens

Some teens develop white spots on their arms that do not tan even with a lot of sun exposure. They're mostly on the tops of the arms and shoulders. Assuming that there is no fungus present in these spots, the most likely diagnosis is pityriasis alba. This is Latin for "scaly white spots." This annoying condition is due to dryness and excess sun exposure. It often starts with mild itching and then progresses to whitish flat spots that just won't tan no matter how much sun you get. We also see these more commonly in women on birth control pills.

Treatment is far from perfect. It consists usually in moisturizing the spots, sometimes with a cortisone lotion if there is any slightly red component of irritation and scale left. If not, a moisturizing sunscreen such as Solbar PF Ultra 50 or Durascreen can be used to solve the dryness and the excess sun exposure problems simultaneously.

The pigment will indeed return; it just takes moisturization and sun avoidance for a while to get the natural-looking skin back.

Sweating Problems

COMPLETELY TREATABLE

Many teens (and adults, for that matter) have tremendous problems with underarm sweating. Sometimes it's so bad that they can virtually never remove their coats in public because of it. The problem is an extremely common one called axillary hyperhidrosis, or excessive underarm sweating. It's due purely to emotional causes. You can prove this to yourself by looking under your arms if you should wake up in the middle of the night. Virtually everyone is dry at this time. That's because the stresses of the day are no longer with us, and the sweating does not occur.

When I was a resident in dermatology, our training director used to demonstrate this fact by asking us to press a palm against a blackboard. Little, if any, wetness resulted, indicating very little moisture or sweating. Then he would ask us to replace our palms on the blackboard and keep them there while he asked us to perform increasingly more difficult mathematical problems. At the end of two minutes of anxious figuring, there were large wet spots on the blackboard where each of us had secreted volumes of sweat during the stress.

It is important to remember that there is a type of sweating that is actually needed by the body. This is the insensible, or unnoticed, water we lose during the daytime. This water loss functions to cool the body and to eliminate certain toxins from the system. However, underarm sweating is not a necessary physiologic process. Underarm sweating, and even palmar sweating for that matter, can be shut down effectively and safely by using a wonderful medicine called Drysol.

Drysol is a concentrated solution of aluminum chloride in alcohol. It's a prescription medicine that can be obtained only on the advice of and consultation with your dermatologist, because he or she must check your underarms for any skin diseases that would prohibit its use. Also, your dermatologist will teach you how to use it and tell you about the mandatory three steps needed to ensure that you get "clothing-dry underarms." This term, coined by Dr. Walter Shelley when he invented Drysol, indicates that while not all sweating disappears from the underarm, enough disappears so that one never has to worry again about removing layers of clothing in public.

Aluminum chloride slows down and even stops eccrine, or watery, sweating in the underarms. To apply, follow these mandatory steps: (1) Your underarms must be completely dry. The medicine cannot be applied immediately after a shower because of residual water in the skin. If necessary, blow-dry the underarms with a hair dryer. (Many patients ask me if I'm kidding when I say this, but I assure you I'm not!) (2) After the medicine is applied, put a six- to eight-inch square piece of plastic wrap in the armpit to protect your nightclothes from the staining properties of Drysol as well as to hold it on the skin so it will be more effective. (3) Wear a T-shirt over your torso during the night to keep the plastic wrap in place. Actually, I advise my patients to mark this T-shirt "DRYSOL," because, with time, the shirt's armpits will be irreparably stained and you will have to change to a new one.

Drysol must be washed off in the morning before clothing is worn. You may think that if leaving it on overnight was effective, possibly leaving it on during the daytime will increase effectiveness, but this is not true. Daytime use is to be avoided because of Drysol's corrosive effects on clothing and the possible irritation of the tender underarm skin.

Besides the fact that it really works, the nicest thing about Drysol is its infrequency of use. While conventional deodorants are applied daily or more often, Drysol is applied only twice on consecutive nights to start, and only once or twice per week thereafter. Fantastic! Sweating stops from the underarms almost instantaneously. This was illustrated quite nicely by a teenage patient of mine named Steve, who came in one day wearing a green sport shirt completely soaked with underarm sweat, all the way down to the belt line. He said that he could no longer go on sweating like this and carry on his daily activities.

I made a quick deal with Steve in order to educate more people about Drysol. He agreed to treat only the right underarm with the medication for two weeks if we could put him on television to teach people about this marvelous medication.

At the end of the second week, Steve returned for the TV tap-
ing with the widest smile I've ever seen. He raised the right arm
high in the air revealing a large objectionable patch of sweat. I was
quite discouraged until he broke into laughter saying, "Don't worry,
Dr. Bark, I switched arms on you!"

Thereupon he raised the left arm and revealed only a tiny,
dime-sized drop of moisture. Steve was very proud, and the video-
tape of his success has helped hundreds of severely sweating
patients cope with their problem.

I have treated hundreds of other people with various sweating
problems, including palm sweating in salespeople, switchboard
operators, and others. Occasionally, it's so bad that these patients
can cup their hands and sweat a small puddle right before my eyes.

One patient, a gun dealer, was about to give up his business
because the sweat from his hands corroded the bluing on gun bar-
rels. After a day or two of Drysol, he went back to work with confidence for the first time in his life. It works even for teenagers whose
feet sweat enough to rot their shoes.

For those who need it, Drysol certainly passes the "Callaway"
test. The Callaway test was originated by one of the greatest dermatologic clinicians and diagnosticians in history, Dr. J. Lamar Callaway
from the Duke University Department of Dermatology, who stated
that a truly effective medicine is the one for which the patient brings
back an empty bottle and says, "Doctor, I've got to have some more
of this stuff!" In other words, a medicine that works.

BODY ODOR

The Drysol technique for stopping perspiration also helps odor
from underarms. To understand this, you must understand a little
about the bacteriology of the underarm skin. There are generally
two types of bacteria on the human skin. The first are gram-positive
bacteria, which normally live on the skin. But some, like staph, can
sometimes infect the skin and cause problems, the chief of which is
body odor. In other words, these bacteria cause smell. The second
type is the gram-negative type. These usually originate in the bowel
areas and are normally on the skin in only very small numbers.
These bacteria normally do not cause an odor.

Deodorants fight body odor by killing off the more common
gram-positive bacteria. This allows the less common gram-negative

bacteria to multiply in the underarms. That's good, because they don't smell. But Drysol is an antiperspirant that actually stops sweating. In most cases Drysol will solve this problem by decreasing wetness, but in some, the malodorous secretions still continue even after Drysol therapy. Dryer underarms mean fewer bacteria, and fewer bacteria usually mean less smell.

A very simple therapy for underarm odor, therefore, is to use a topical antibiotic that cuts down on the numbers of gram-positive bacteria. While most "deodorant soaps" have antibacterial properties, they are not strong enough for difficult cases. In such situations, topical antibiotics such as neomycin can help amazingly. Ask your dermatologist about this and other antibiotics such as topical cleocin, erythromycin, and garamycin.

Also, be aware that there are very rare diseases of metabolism, in which certain protein building blocks called amino acids may be present in excess. Usually these people have this body odor problem early in life. If this is the case, as it seems to be in some kids, it is necessary to have some tests done of their protein system, to make sure that all is normal.

FAILURE TO SWEAT

Occasionally in practice we encounter a patient who has very, very dry skin and does not perspire. Some of these people nearly pass out in what is not excessive heat for a normal person. Sometimes this causes great physical stress, with a very rapid pulse and extreme discomfort. Some of these people have complete or nearly complete absence of sweat glands, a disorder called congenital anhidrotic ectodermal defect. This condition leaves the victim without one of the body's most important cooling mechanisms, that of evaporative sweating. Without this major air-conditioning device, tolerance for heat is almost nil. These people can have heat strokes in even mildly elevated temperatures.

It's vital for such patients to visit a dermatologist skilled in the evaluation of this condition, so that the presence or absence of sweat glands and their normal function can be documented. If a congenital anhidrotic ectodermal defect is confirmed, then the patient will need to avoid hot environments at all costs. As yet, we have no other therapy for the condition.

ᑦattoos

Lasers may well be the best way to remove large tattoos. If you're looking for a reputable specialist who does a certain medical procedure in your area, always be sure to call the local medical society and the local university's department of dermatology if there's one nearby. One or the other should be able to refer you. If not, you may write the American Academy of Dermatology at:

American Academy of Dermatology
PO Box 4014
Schaumburg, IL 60168-4014

Don't expect a "no-scar result," however, with any means of tattoo removal. That pigment is deep within the dermis, or second layer of the skin, and it's tough to get out. The laser's light is so powerful that when it strikes the pigment in the tattoo area, the pigment is vaporized into smoke immediately. But the heat of the procedure does induce some scarring, just as would a third-degree burn in the same area.

Tinea Versicolor

Often, patients develop whitish spots on their shoulders and chests. At first they start out small and few, over the upper torso. They begin as just dry white patches and then turn whiter than the surrounding skin. This is a fungus infection called tinea versicolor (TV). Tinea versicolor is Latin for "many-colored fungus." The name comes from the fact that, during the summertime, the fungus prohibits tanning. To do this it secretes an acid that shuts down the pigment cells in the skin. Occasionally, during the wintertime, they can even look darker than the surrounding skin. As yet, we don't understand exactly why the darker phase occurs. Some scaling accompanies these discolored spots, but frequently there are very few symptoms.

The TV fungus is usually caught by direct or indirect contact with someone else who has had it. That is, one can contract the spores of the fungus by using someone else's towel in gym class, by trying on a blouse at a department store after an infected person has done the same and deposited some of the spores, or, of course, by direct skin-to-skin contact.

There appears to be a large factor of individual susceptibility, however, since not all those who have contact with the fungus get the disease. Some people obviously have a natural resistance. Fungus grows very high up on the skin layers so that it is not really attacked by the body's usually efficient systems of eliminating infections. Even more important, the fungus spores lodge down inside the hair follicles and can spread back onto the skin after local treatments have knocked out all the surface fungus. This fact was amply demonstrated several years ago when electron microscope pictures of a hair follicle revealed the spores deep below the surface. It was then that we dermatologists found out why we had such little success in treating this stubborn problem.

NEW TREATMENTS

Since that time, however, we have developed a few new bullets for our treatment gun, which can help tremendously. One of these was the recent discovery that propylene glycol, a common solvent used to dilute and mix other dermatologic medications, actually kills this fungus. While this medication is occasionally slightly irritating, it's extremely safe to use and should be relatively cheap to have mixed up by one's pharmacist on the prescription of a dermatologist. Prior to the advent of propylene glycol therapy we used a very foul-smelling topical sulfur lotion called selenium sulfide, which was applied and left on for a considerable length of time. The stuff was so rotten-smelling that it would not only obliterate one's fungus but would also blow away one's relatives if they were anywhere nearby! Thankfully, those days are now passing with the advent of new treatment preparations for this disease. We still use sulfur in a minor way, in sulfur-containing soaps, which are effective in preventing a recurrence of the fungus for several months after treatment.

Even more recently two new antifungal medicines have been found to be extremely effective in wiping out this long-term nuisance. They are ketoconazole (Nizoral) and Sporonox, newly introduced oral antifungals that treat TV very easily. One has to take the pills only once a month for a year to rid oneself of this problem. There have been rare cases of liver irritation with ketoconazole, however, so ask your dermatologist to explain all possible side effects of the drug. He or she may want you to get occasional lab tests to check the status of your liver while you are under treatment for the fungus. Take careful note that although Nizoral and Sporonox are very effective in TV, they are not FDA-approved for this disease. Many dermatologists will not use them for this indication. I do, but only after carefully informing the patient of any possible risks.

When the fungus is gone and the pigment suppressor chemical is no longer secreted, the color cells will again turn on their production of normal pigment and the skin will return to its usual shade. It may take some months for the pigment to return, so be patient. If there is any trouble retanning, one should see one's dermatologist again for further information and to make sure that one doesn't have either a recurrence of the disease or some other problem associated with lack of pigment.

Tylosis

CUT HOSIERY BILLS—
CURE YOUR ROUGH HEELS

The scaly heel problem, called tylosis, is a real annoyance to women because the scaly areas on the heels can crack, bleed, and even run hosiery. While the problem occasionally has another cause, such as a fungus or an allergic contact dermatitis, it's more usually the result of severe dryness on the feet, especially the thick heel areas. There are even inherited cases that are quite extreme.

There are treatments for this problem, such as conventional moisturizers, soaks of various kinds, and over-the-counter medicines, but over the years, I've found a regimen that works better for my patients than any other I've ever tried. Ask your doctor for prescriptions for the two medicines, but I think you'll find it well worth the price of the office call. You may have to do this whole procedure only two to three times weekly to keep smoother feet.

It goes like this: Soak your feet in warm, clear tap water for about twenty to thirty minutes at night. Pat your feet dry, and apply a good layer of Keralyt gel (one of the prescription items) over the affected areas. Then cover each of your feet with a plastic bag, followed by a sock over the bag. You should not tape the bag down; just cover it with a sock. Leave this occlusive bandage on all night. Be careful not to slip with the plastic bags on your feet. Bags and carpets are a slippery combination.

In the morning, take off the bags and wipe the sweat, dead skin cells, and remaining medicine off your feet. Then apply a good layer of LacHydrin lotion (the other prescription medicine).

Keep in mind that heels that have deep, tender, and/or bleeding splits or fissures may need internal antibiotics to encourage them to heal. Your dermatologist will tell you if he thinks this will help.

If you follow the above program regularly, I'm fairly certain that you won't have much of a problem with feet looking more like elephant hide than like skin. Remember, you must see your doctor for this treatment, but it's worth it.

$\mathcal{W}arts$

Childhood warts are the bane of the dermatologist's existence. These nasty growths, called verruca vulgaris, are caused by the minuscule human papilloma virus.

The fact that they are caused by a virus means they are contagious. One of the most annoying problems in the office practice of dermatology is that pediatricians, family physicians, and other primary care doctors often advise that the lesions will fade and heal completely on their own. While this may indeed be true in an isolated circumstance, read on before you decide to treat them with "watchful waiting."

A patient of mine I'll call Terry was entering the all-important third year of medical school when students get their first "hands-on" experience. But poor Terry couldn't conceive of it with his hands; we counted over 200 warts on his palms.

He told me a long and classic story about the development of warts. "When I was about seven years old," he said, "I only had one wart on my wrist, but within the next few months, several new baby warts had developed around it. I was a real picker, Doc, and that seemed to spread them and make the warts multiply. I feel very embarrassed about examining patients with my hands like this, and I wondered what you could do."

Terry had waited too long. Now the job of removing his warts was a mammoth task instead of a minor inconvenience. The fact is that, while an isolated wart may indeed resolve, seemingly by magic (probably an immune or protective reaction by the body), others may develop from the spread of the virus. That's the reason I try to lecture to pediatricians constantly about the natural history of warts. I encourage them to treat the warts or refer them for treatment earlier so that the final job is not such a colossal one. Ideally, I like to treat children before they can pick or chew at their warts and spread them around as Terry had done. I have actually seen children with hundreds of facial warts caused by biting finger warts.

While an individual wart could be expected to go away on its own over a certain length of time (usually months to years), it is shedding virus constantly and possibly causing baby warts to develop that will also need to be treated. The key is, don't wait. Get your child to a dermatologist for treatment.

There is no magic age at which warts will resolve. If your family practitioner or pediatrician cannot treat warts, then consult a dermatologist. Dermatologists can treat the problem in many different ways, which we'll discuss later in this chapter.

You should know that the virus, although living in the warts, is technically on the body; it is not in the body or in the bloodstream.

Warts do not have "roots." This concept of warts growing like trees and plants is utter nonsense! The terminology got started long ago when scraped-off warts revealed a velvety rootlike surface below. Also, if you look down on a wart, you can see small dots in the surface of the wart which the old-timers called "seeds." But there are no seeds or roots in warts. The dots you see are merely thrombosed, or plugged, capillaries which feed the surface of the wart. Warts do not grow down into other tissues. In fact, each and every wart is a simple epidermal growth. That is, it grows in the most superficial layer of skin and never penetrates the dermis or second layer of skin. That's why they don't scar if they're removed carefully and gently.

BEST TREATMENTS

There are about as many treatments for warts as there are patients who have them, and there is no one perfect treatment. The key words in wart therapy are "first do no harm," the physician's prime imperative. In short, when taking off warts, physicians don't want to cause a scar or mark that looks worse than the wart did or that lasts longer than the wart might have lasted. That's why we've largely abandoned treatments that burn off or cut off warts because of the scar left behind.

These days we rely on treatments that, although not uniformly successful the first time, can remove a wart dependably in most cases if the follow-up is adequate. Among these techniques is the application of various chemicals and/or acids to the wart surface in order to scale it off slowly. Many "wart removers" are available over the counter. They are much less effective than your doctor's treatments.

A seven-year-old boy named Jerry came in one day, and his mother said that the large wart on his foot was finally going away under the influence of an over-the-counter substance. Since that was about the first time I had ever heard that a wart actually was making progress with this preparation, I was anxious to see the spot. When I pulled off Jerry's sock, I saw a large blistered heel wart with redness and tenderness almost up to his ankle! What had happened was immediately apparent. My one and only witnessed cure of this wart with this over-the-counter medicine occurred because Jerry had gotten allergic to this medicine, not because it actually worked in its intended manner. This severe allergic reaction had blown the wart away (although quite painfully).

A popular way to remove warts is by the use of cryosurgery. This literally means "surgery with cold." In this technique, the skin is sprayed lightly with liquid nitrogen at the remarkable temperature of minus 196° C. Believe me, that's even colder than our average Lexington winter! This freezing method makes a small split or blister just below the wart. As the blister arises, the wart is pushed upward. Then the blister falls off, and if all parts of the wart were frozen adequately, the wart falls off with the blister top. Occasionally, with larger lesions, the technique has to be repeated several times at two- to three-week intervals.

But it's not all that easy with the freezing treatment. The freezing of small parts of the skin creates a miniature case of frostbite, and that hurts! A year or two ago a little red-haired six-year-old was trying to be a very brave soldier while I froze his huge finger warts. As I froze two or three of his larger warts, I could see tears forming, then I heard a plaintive little cry, and finally he looked up at me and growled, "You'd better stop it or I'm gonna call the police!"

Well, we froze the warts on that occasion and on one other and he did fine, without scars, but I'll never forget his warning. By the way, the police never came.

DIET, VITAMINS, AND WARTS

As a viral disease, warts can attack anyone who has skin, regardless of his or her diet. They recur sometimes because this virus may have already spread to other areas.

There is no magic vitamin or pill you can take to get rid of warts. Rubbing them with vitamin E has no value whatsoever. The vitamin E therapy brings up a point, however: Vitamin E seems to be the new folk remedy that has replaced some of the other old wives' tales used for years to treat warts.

Some of these are quite interesting. I have collected dozens of folk remedies for warts, including the following:

> Rub the wart with a potato; then bury the potato in the backyard.
>
> Ask your grandmother to buy your wart for a penny or a nickel (inflation has probably raised this to at least a quarter by now!).
>
> Touch the warts with a dishrag; then bury the rag under the front steps.
>
> Tie one knot in a string for each wart, and then drop the string over your shoulder by the light of a full moon.
>
> Rub the wart with a piece of chalk (amazingly enough, this technique is actually practiced by more than one reputable dermatologist).
>
> Paint stale stump water on the wart.
>
> Rub the juice from a milkweed on the wart.
>
> Have a hypnotist "exorcize" the wart.

All these techniques are accompanied by reports that on occasion they actually do work. This is the "placebo effect" in wart therapy: It is well known that in rare instances just the suggestion that a medicine will work actually brings on resolution of the lesion.

Obviously, when the placebo effect works in warts, something has happened chemically to remove it, but as yet, no one knows what that something is. It may be a low-grade allergic reaction to the wart tissue itself.

What we really need is a wart vaccine. However, this tiny virus cannot yet be cultured or grown outside the human body, so this is, as yet, not possible. Work proceeds in this direction, however. Some investigators have derived a vaccine by grinding up wart tissue and administering it by injection, but other researchers warn that this may be a very dangerous practice. You see, the wart virus is a DNA virus, and DNA is that stuff that controls all cell mechanisms. No one wants extra DNA in his or her system since it might be possible that it could cause cancers and/or other problems.

FINGERNAIL WARTS

Patients often complain about warts growing at or near the edges of the fingernails. These are some of the most difficult warts to clear up. In fact, some patients try to "do their own surgery," by using nail clippers and cuticle nippers to cut away the warty skin. First of all, cuticle clippers should never be used. Cutting into these warts may cause localized infection. You also get wart virus on the clippers and may spread warts around if you use them in other areas. And worse yet, anyone who uses your clippers can get them. I've seen them spread like wildfire through whole families by this route. The difficulty with warts around the nails (periungual warts) is that the virus hides under the free edge of the nail and is almost impossible to get rid of by freezing in this location. Often, freezing is used to reduce the size of the warts so that other therapies can be used.

For periungual warts (the most difficult to treat anywhere), I have found very little that is completely effective. One of the best agents used for this process is squaric acid. This compound is a type of topically, or surface-applied, medicine that is highly allergenic. That is, the body very easily forms an allergic reaction to it in much the same way it reacts to poison ivy. The medicine is applied in very dilute form to a "sensitization area" (such as the inside of the arm), by the dermatologist or the doctor's staff under an aluminum patch that is left on for about twenty-four hours. Soon the patch-tested area reacts, gets red, and itches. Then the treatment period starts. A small amount of squaric acid in cream form is applied to the warts and is poked in gently with a wooden toothpick. This activates an allergic reaction in and around the wart, and intense inflammation in the area calls out the body's immune system and very effectively wipes out the wart.

It may take several months, including multiple applications, to cause the allergy, but after it occurs, treatment of the warts is a simple process of applying the medicine repeatedly.

PLANTAR (SOLE) WARTS

Some dermatologists say that they would rather see a minor case of skin cancer than a plantar wart (a wart on the bottom of the foot). Plantar warts are ordinary skin warts that have grown on the sole. The term "plantar"" refers to the plantar, or bottom, surface of the foot as opposed to the volar, or top surface. It has nothing to do with the word "planter." These warts are tough to get rid of because they are pushed into the skin rather than being allowed to grow out above the skin of the foot. They do not have roots that grow into or around bones, or penetrate the actual foot substance. They are surface growths that are just pushed inward. But since they are located in a weight-bearing area, they can be very painful and are difficult to treat.

Cryosurgery cannot be used on the foot in most instances because it's too painful and much less effective in this particular location, because the skin is so thick in the foot area. A blister could be produced in such skin, but only with a heroic freeze that would at least temporarily disable the patient, so I do not advise freezing warts on the thick weight-bearing skin of the soles. It is a different matter on the insteps and undersurfaces of the toes, however, since that skin is thinner and can be frozen lightly enough to accomplish the purpose of curing the wart without disabling the patient.

X-ray therapy has been used very effectively in the treatment of plantar warts. While X-ray therapy often does work in up to 85 percent of single warts, treatment is reserved only for the most recalcitrant or stubborn single warts.

Obviously, one worries about the long-term effects of radiation on the bones and inner tissues of the foot, such as cancer, ulcers, and scarring. But a study in the dermatologic literature of some 7,000 patients showed X-ray treatment to be extremely safe therapy. However, most dermatologists have given up this treatment because having an X-ray unit in their offices hugely increases their liability insurance.

Let me warn you strongly against having surgery on the bottom of the foot. This almost always causes a permanent scar, which can actually hurt more than the original wart because of pressure exerted upon it while walking. The same is true for laser therapy for warts on the bottom of the feet. This can cause a prolonged period of disability during healing, and potential scarring can result.

So we turn to other therapies for these stubborn warts on the soles. Among the old-fashioned but effective remedies for plantar warts is a substance called podophyllin. Podophyllin is a plant resin which kills the rapidly multiplying skin cells that contain the wart virus. Its irritating action works on plantar warts only when it is bandaged onto the wart for extended times (sometimes ten to fourteen days). Used in this way, it can effectively eliminate a wart if the pain is not too disagreeable. Be very careful to ask your doctor how much pain might be involved. If you need to step on the brake of your car firmly, you could have an accident if the pain prevents you from doing so, or it could interfere with your job if you must spend a lot of time on your feet.

After the initial podophyllin treatment, which removes the body of the wart, I use a technique employing a 3-percent solution of a substance called glutaraldehyde. In this technique, the patient soaks a small part of a cotton ball with the solution and tapes it onto the warty area for fifteen minutes twice daily. Glutaraldehyde kills the cells harboring the wart virus, and sooner or later the wart grows up and out and off of the skin. This is one of the few techniques that is successful in removing large, multiple, or mosaic plantar warts. Sometimes the wart is covered with a plaster of salicylic acid, which helps the medicine penetrate into the wart.

During this treatment your dermatologist will see you every few weeks to pare down the superficial dead skin and check to see if there is any residual wart. You will then be told if you need to continue the treatment.

The glutaraldehyde technique has defeated the largest wart I have ever seen, a huge three-by-five-inch wart that covered nearly the entire sole. The patient, Judy, who had this huge wart had been treated with every known therapy, including cryosurgery, the pain of which I decided to risk because of the disability caused by this monster wart. She couldn't walk anyway, so in this case the blisters could not be any more painful. Since she had put up with this wart since she was a toddler, she was willing to try anything. That's when I decided to try the formalin therapy suggested by a dermatologist friend from Tallahassee. *Note well:* Glutaraldehyde is poisonous if taken internally. Do not make any attempt to smell this medicine because it is quite irritating to the nasal passages. Take special precautions to keep this and all medicines out of the reach of your children. You can use it on your children safely, but don't let the bottle get into their hands. This technique should be used only when supervised by a dermatologist skilled in its use.

After she was put on the glutaraldehyde therapy, Judy disappeared from my office until approximately a year later. When she came back for me to check another skin problem, I asked her if I could take a look at her wart. She grinned coyly and took off her shoe. I was flabbergasted. The only trace that there had ever been a wart in the area was a small scar where she had attempted to have the wart cut off years before I treated her. She said that her wart resolved slowly over several months of using this special therapy. We were both thrilled and amazed at this incredible result.

I want to stress that warts occur on the bottom of the feet only because people go barefoot. In fact, that may be the only way people catch them. Therefore, even at home, and certainly in public places such as swimming pools, hotels, and gymnasium locker rooms, do not go barefoot. The best protection against contracting warts in pool areas or gyms is to wear rubber thongs, or "flip-flops." They can stop the skin from picking up this nuisance virus. If you already have plantar warts and want to avoid spreading them to the other members of your family, you should not only wear flops in the showers in your house, but you should scrub the tub with a chlorine cleanser following each use. Otherwise, there may be more than one member of your family seeking dermatologic care for plantar warts.

One other newer therapy for isolated plantar warts must be mentioned, because it is so effective in eliminating them. This technique is called bleomycin injection. Bleomycin is a drug used to treat certain cancers. When injected in tiny amounts under plantar warts, irritation is produced that sheds the wart over the next three weeks or so. Often, we inject warts with bleomycin and then see the patient back in two weeks or so to pare down the dead warty skin and examine the base of the wart to see if any further treatment is needed. Most of the time a single injection can clear the wart permanently. Two cautions about the use of bleomycin in wart therapy. First, the injection of a substance into the tight tissues of the bottom of the foot is *painful*. And while the pain is short-lived, it is significant. Second, bleomycin, as of this writing, is *not* approved by the FDA for use in warts. It is something that you and your dermatologist must discuss in detail, because it *is* accepted practice to use drugs in other-than-approved uses. Just so you and your dermatologist have this clearly understood.

FRUSTRATING FACIAL WARTS

One of the other more frustrating types of warts are flat warts on the face. Often these warts are misdiagnosed by the patients as "acne" or other conditions. In reality, they are one of the many types of wart virus infections of the facial skin, forming flat-topped bumps that are best visible in tangential or side-lighting. Recently, there have been good reports on 5-fluorouracil (5-FU) cream, a medicine used in the elderly to remove premalignant sunspots. It is also reliable for removing flat warts on the face. It does this by slowing the multiplication of the wart-containing cells and by inducing irritation in the warts themselves. This cream, while slightly irritating to the skin, does a fine job in many instances. Ask your doctor about it. When using this medicine, stay out of the sun. This drug is made more potent and irritating by the sun's rays. If you get an irritation instead of a cure from it, call your doctor. Sometimes we combine Efudex treatment with a vitamin A acid compound called Retin-A, which was designed to be used in acne. It enhances the penetration of the Efudex and, while causing significantly greater irritation, it also enhances the cure rate of flat warts.

GENITAL WARTS

One of the most troubling problems for women is the problem of genital warts. Naturally, men get them too, but the most important thing for patients to realize is that viral warts grow like wildfire on some patients, absolutely defying the doctor's every attempt to annihilate them. In the vaginal area, because of the natural wetness, the nasty virus spreads with even greater alacrity.

Researchers have found that there are at least forty different types of wart virus. Some of these types smolder along for years, slowly decreasing the amount of infectious virus they secrete. Apparently, while they're becoming less and less infectious, they are also, unfortunately, becoming associated more and more with cancer in the vulvar area. That is, these long-term lesions are worrying researchers in the field that they may some day cause cancer. That's why, for the most part, we advise women to get these off as soon as practical. These facts aside, however, you wouldn't want your husband to show up with warts on his genitals, so you really should have them removed.

More important, some virologists feel that laryngeal papillomas, small growths on the vocal cords, may be caused by contacting wart virus in the mother's birth canal during delivery. For that reason alone, vaginal warts should be treated.

PENILE WARTS

Warts on the genitals are called venereal warts. In every single case, because of their contagious nature, they should be treated. It's not easy, and even painful at times, but if you value protecting your sex contacts from them, have your skin doctor treat them.

The treatments for warts include podophyllin, electrocautery, cryosurgery, conventional surgery, and laser surgery. Podophyllin is a plant resin that irritates the warts off your skin—if you're lucky! Occasionally, it causes so much irritation that cortisone medications are necessary to cool down the area. This medicine is dangerous from this standpoint and should never be dispensed by prescription for the patient's use. It's always put on in the doctor's office. The doctor will give you very specific instructions on washing it off in four to eight hours. Do this exactly as your doctor instructs.

Recently, a medicine called Condylox has been released for home use by patients for their warts. Condylox is the active ingredient in podophyllin. This small and expensive bottle of medicine contains a small applicator and directions for applying it directly and only to the wart in a prescribed manner. You must get these instructions directly from the dermatologist and make sure that he or she marks the lesions to be treated so that you are not choosing the spots. The dermatologist knows what warts look like—you may not, and may treat something that has no bearing on warts at all. So have the spots you are to treat marked first, before embarking on a program of treatment with Condylox.

Electrocautery is rarely used, due to scarring. Burning off warts went out with the ancients, and certainly should not be used on one of the most important and tender areas of the body.

Cryosurgery (freezing the wart off with liquid nitrogen) is my favorite choice for genital warts. It makes a small scab out of the wart, which will drop off in a week or two. Of course, the areas should be checked as often as possible to guard against recurrences. Recurrent small warts should be refrozen as soon as you notice them. This treatment stings a bit but is very effective.

Conventional scalpel removal of warts is usually avoided because of scarring.

Laser treatment of warts is now becoming popular because of the great ability of the laser light to virtually vaporize tissue on contact. You'll hear a lot more about this technique in the future.

Large warts give concern, because certain large warts can have skin cancer in their bases. Any large wart, therefore, should be treated as soon as possible, and if it is recurrent, a biopsy should be performed to check for this disease.

WARTS AND CANCER

Common skin warts that we are apt to see on our children never turn into skin cancer. I repeat, common warts never turn into skin cancer. Two cases in which there is some suspicion that warts may be related to skin cancer both relate to genital warts, and we will talk more about those elsewhere.

The real problem is that patients don't have the training to tell the difference between warts, moles, and skin cancers. That's why the American Cancer Society advises examination in any case where there's concern. The bottom line is that you probably don't have the expertise to tell the difference. Even dermatologists occasionally biopsy bumps that look strange and eventually turn out to be only warts. The "take-home" message is that you wouldn't want to assume that a skin cancer was a wart and not get it treated in time. When in doubt, see a skin expert!

Wrinkles

MOISTURIZERS

If we read the lay magazines, beauty magazines, and other publications, we are told constantly to moisturize our skin to prevent or minimize wrinkling. Can moisturizer really prevent wrinkles? Not really. Only sun avoidance prevents wrinkles. Moisturizers only soften the superficial skin a little, making it feel slightly better and more supple. The wrinkles just laugh at the stuff. You should also realize that some of the least expensive moisturizers work best. Some, such as Moisturel and Lubriderm, actually do a better job of moisturizing the skin without ill effects (such as acne cosmetica, allergies, and irritation) than the very expensive ones.

SMOKING—A CAUSE OF WRINKLES?

Several years ago a study was published stating you could tell the side on which a woman held her cigarette while smoking by the severity of wrinkles on that side. The authors maintained that this may be due to squinting as smoke wafts by the eyes. They also considered the possibility that some noxious chemical might be causing the skin to wrinkle.

When researchers sought to reproduce the study, it was shown to be, for the most part, invalid. I can only say in my experience as a clinician seeing thousands of women for all sorts of skin problems, I think that smoking women are more severely and more coarsely wrinkled than are nonsmokers.

COLLAGEN TREATMENTS

One of the most effective ways to handle wrinkles of a minor type is an injectable form of collagen. That, as you remember, is what comprises the support network of the skin. The Collagen Corporation

230

has refined a technique for injecting the components of skin into a defect or depressed spot, such as a forehead wrinkle, where the material actually reassembles itself into near-human collagen. The medicine is called Zyderm, it is FDA approved, and can work wonders.

There are other ways to smooth aging, wrinkled skin. Dermabrasion is the superficial sanding off of the upper two layers of the facial skin. A chemical peel refers to an acid treatment of the same layers of the skin. Both procedures are done to alleviate scarring and minor wrinkles in the facial skin. Talk to your dermatologist and/or plastic surgeon about obtaining the procedures, if they are warranted.

Index

Chin-strap acne, 33
Chocolate, and acne, 15-16
Chronic epilation, 109
Cimetidine, 19
Claritin, and psoriasis, 168
Clinique Cosmetics, 35
    Pore Minimizer Makeup, 154
Cold sores, 116-18
Collagen:
    implants, 27-28
    injection, 28
        complications of, 29-30
    and wrinkles, 230
Color correction foundation, 56
Comedo extractor, 31-32
Complex 15, 114
Condylox, 228
Congenital melanocytic nevi, 51
Contact urticaria syndrome,
        113-14
Cooling of the skin, 2
Cornrow hair loss, 60-61
    darker spots, 61-62
Corns, 66
Cornstarch powders, and baby
        skin, 48
Cortisone:
    and alopecia areata, 107-8
    and eczema, 77
    and psoriasis, 163, 164
Cortisone injections, 30
Cosmetic allergies, 37-41
    lipstick rashes, 38-39
    nickel allergies, 39-41
Cosmetics:
    and acne, 34-35
    eye infections from, 81-82
    and skin, 67
    and skin cancer, 181
Covermark Cosmetics, 54
Croton oil, 106
Cryocurettage method, seborrhiec
        keratoses, 174
Cryosurgery:
    and seborrhiec keratoses, 174-75

and squamous cell carcinoma
        (SCCA), 187-88
    and warts, 224, 229
Cuticle, 84-85
Cystic acne, and Accutane, 12-13
Cysts, 68

D

Dandruff, 69-71
Dark circles under the eyes, 82
Demodex, 179
De Morgan's spots, 44
Depilatories, 110
Dermablend, 54-55
Dermabrasion, 25-27, 30
    cost of, 26
Dermatopathic lymphadenopathy,
        33-34
Diet:
    and acne, 15-16
    and breast skin cysts, 68
    and warts, 221-23
Dihydrotestosterone (DHT), 94
Dihydroxyacetone, 200
Dimethylglyoxine (DMG) kit,
        40-41
Diprolene lotion, 164
Dove soap, and eczema, 79
Dove Unscented, and hand
        eczema, 112
Drithocreme, 169
Dritho-Scalp, 169
Dry skin, 72-76
    genesis of, 72-75
    heritability of, 75-76
    and humidifiers, 75
    moisturizers, 74-75
    nummular eczema, 75
    winter itch, 72
    xerosis, 72-74
Drysol, 211-14
Durascreen 30, 197
Dysplastic nevus syndrome, 192